The Orphan's Father

The Orphan's Father

Ayurveda: Curing Modern Medicine's
Abandoned Diseases

Dr. Narasimham V. Jammi

ISBN 13: 978-93-90976-78-2
ISBN 10: 93-90976-78-2

Printed in India and published by BUUKS.

Dedication

*I dedicate this book to Sri 1008 Satyatma Tirtha Swamiji, Peethadipati,
Sri Uttaradi Matha, India; without whose blessings and inspiration, I would not have
had the fortitude to take on the rather overwhelming task of managing several projects
and responsibilities. His Holiness is singularly responsible for all that I am today.*

Table of Contents

Foreword   ix

About the Author   xi

Chapter 1   Churning of the Oceans: The Origins of Ayurveda   1

Chapter 2   Sushruta and the Nose Job: Heroes of Ayurveda   12

Chapter 3   Heavy, Heavy Fuel: Myths Associated with
Raw Materials, Metals, and Minerals   26

Chapter 4   The Hare and the Tortoise: Myths about the
Slow Action of Ayurvedic Medicines   40

Chapter 5   The Gourmand's Curse: Myths Associated
with Dietary Practices in Ayurveda   53

Chapter 6   A Streetcar Named Desire: The Role of Ayurveda in
Reproductive Health, Childbirth and the Baby's Early
Years   73

Chapter 7   Kapil Dev, an All-Rounder Par Excellence:
The 360-Degree Holistic System that is Ayurveda   93

Chapter 8   Beauty is Not Skin Deep: Beauty Regimens in
Ayurveda versus Cosmetic Cover-Ups   110

Chapter 9   International Yoga Day: Why Yoga is an Important
Aspect of Ayurveda   127

Foreword

WHY THIS BOOK?

As is painfully evident from the COVID-19 pandemic, it is a given that most people will be exposed to the virus. Being able to fight off the virus without falling sick or maybe just a mild illness will be the ideal situation. However, many people have succumbed to the disease. But a far greater number of people have actually recovered without falling seriously ill. What is the difference between these two sets of people? If you guessed - their immunity; then you'd be 100 percent on the money! The only way to build immunity (other than a vaccine, which is very specific to one particular disease) is over the long term, by eating right, exercising regularly, and having the right supplements. Enter Ayurveda to the rescue! This is where Ayurveda scores over other systems. Why? Because the right diet, appropriate exercise, and healthy supplements (read Ayurvedic *rasayanas*) are the only solution to promote and maintain wellness. I'd rather spend my time and efforts in building my immunity and maintaining my wellness than waste my hard-earned money on fighting off an illness by whichever 'pathy.' It is this information that I want to communicate to the reader without spending too much time on esoteric stuff. This book is NOT a technical treatise. It is, however, a quick, short peep through the keyhole into the wondrous world of Ayurveda.

About the Author

A SCIENTIST WITH a PhD in Biological Chemistry (University of Utah, Salt Lake City) and postdoctoral experience in Molecular Pharmacology (Stanford University), Dr. Narasimham Jammi was brought up in an environment filled with a steady diet of Ayurvedic thought processes. Though not formally trained in Ayurveda, Dr. Narasimham Jammi has been learning Ayurveda for the last 12 years from his father, who himself learned from his grandfather, who learned from his great grandfather. Adopting Ayurveda and avoiding allopathy as much as possible has made a massive difference to his quality of life, and the improvements in his health quotient (he calls it the H.Q.) have been immense. He hopes this book will serve to clarify various doubts that readers may have about Ayurveda. Having been part of the Ayurveda setup for four generations (nearly 125 years), Jammi believes that Ayurveda has a lot to give to the world in the present situation. He advocates the use of Ayurveda wherever possible, and is actively engaged in understanding the molecular mechanisms of various Ayurvedic formulations. He has pursued research on many wonderful ayurvedic entities in collaboration with various research institutes like Indian Institute of Technology (IIT)-Delhi; Tata Memorial Advanced Centre for Treatment and Research in Cancer (ACTREC), Mumbai; University of Madras, Chennai; Delhi Pharmaceutical Sciences and Research University (DPSRU), Delhi; and Asthagiri Research Foundation, Chennai. His goal is to make sure that Ayurveda is adopted as part of everyone's lifestyle, and he is on a mission to do this using various forums. *The Orphan's Father* is one such attempt to achieve that goal.

CHAPTER 1

Churning of the Oceans:
The Origins of Ayurveda

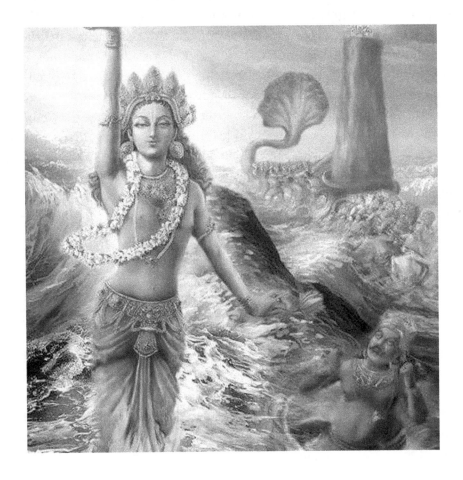

I DIDN'T KNOW it then, but I was just about to hear a story that would go on to play a huge role in my life.

It was a balmy evening in May, and we were over at my grandparents' house in Adyar in Chennai. We were bang in the middle of our summer vacations—and back then, what with all of us cousins together, that typically meant a raucous evening ahead! This day was no different. We had devised a thrilling game that involved a lot of yelling and chasing each other around the house. At one point, I had grabbed a bedsheet that was hanging on the line and had tossed it at my cousin to slow him down. But of course, once he got over the initial surprise, he just grabbed the sheet and continued chasing me with it. Before we knew it, we were each holding on to one side of the bedsheet and pulling with all our might. What's more, our younger siblings and cousins had finally caught up, and they started taking sides in this impromptu tug of war. This went on for a few minutes until . . . there was an almighty *RIIIPPP* and the bedsheet split right down the middle! To make matters worse, my cousin lost his balance and collided with a vase, taking it down with him. We knew we were in big trouble.

Sure enough, the crash brought my mother and my aunt rushing in from another room. As is often the case with grown-ups, they were least interested in knowing who started it! We were all handed out severe punishments and dire warnings about what they would do to us if they heard another peep from us for the rest of the day. Having had first-hand knowledge about the fallouts of neglecting such warnings, we decided it would be a good idea to lay low for a while. We grabbed a textbook each and settled down, not even daring to talk to one another. Mamma, our softhearted grandmother, felt bad at our sorry plight. Soon, we heard the soft clink of her bangles and turned to see her standing there, armed with a plateful of mangos.

'You should be careful when you do that, you know,' she said in her gentle voice as she came in and sat down on the wooden armchair in one corner of the room. 'That tug of war, you never know what will come out of it.'

Cheered by the sight of those juicy mango slices, we set our books aside. We sidled up to her and sat cross-legged around the chair on the cool red floor. 'What do you mean?' I asked, sensing a story coming.

'Well, the Devatas did something like this eons ago—but first, they had to put in a lot of effort to prepare for it. Let me tell you about the Samudra Manthana . . .'

Samudra Manthana

It all began at a time when the Devatas were at the peak of their glory. Indra, the ruler of the realms, was resplendent in his power and might—and he had transfused his energy and abilities to all the Devatas in his realm. One day, Indra set out on his elephant to tour his realm. On the way, he met the renowned sage, Durvasa. Sage Durvasa was a learned and kind-hearted rishi—but he was a man who was not to be crossed, for he had a quick temper too. Sage Durvasa was very happy to see Lord Indra in all his splendor, so he greeted him with a garland. Lord Indra, in a momentary lapse of propriety, placed the garland on his elephant's trunk, who in turn threw it upon the ground. This ignited Durvasa's anger. Offended at having his gift thus dismissed, he cursed Lord Indra and proclaimed that he would soon lose all his splendor until he had nothing left to be the lord of. This marked the beginning of the Devatas' downfall. Sensing their weakness, the Asuras saw their opportunity and started encroaching upon their kingdom. Before long, the scales had tilted, and the Asuras had become more powerful, while the Devatas were at an all-time low.

In desperation, Lord Indra approached Lord Brahma, the Creator, and asked for his help. Lord Brahma then suggested that they go to Lord Vishnu, the Supreme Being. They invoked Lord Vishnu and begged for his help. Lord Vishnu listened to the Devatas and agreed to come to their aid. He told them of the 'amrita' —the nectar of immortality—that lies beneath the milky ocean, Kshirasagara. But he warned them that obtaining it would not be easy. They would need to churn the ocean until the amrita came out.

The Devatas were aghast at the idea of churning the vast expanse of the ocean. But Lord Vishnu helped them to look beyond their limitations and told them how it could be done. He told them that they would first need to seek out the right herbs and plants to put into the ocean to ensure that the right things came out. So that's what the Devatas did. Some believe that this is the very first example of Ayurveda in practice.

Next, Lord Vishnu advised the Devatas to approach the Asuras and ask for their help, because a task of this magnitude would not be possible to achieve alone. So, Lord Indra went to the Asuras, but understandably, they turned him down. In order to get them to cooperate, Lord Indra negotiated with the Asuras and promised to split everything that came out of the ocean. On hearing this, the Asuras finally agreed.

After this, the Devatas were to look for a churning rod and a rope large enough to churn an entire ocean. The Devatas were stumped. That's when Lord Vishnu directed their attention to the Mandara Parvata—a mountain that was large enough to function as a churning rod. But try as they might, the Devatas were unable to move the Mandara Parvata even by a single inch. They turned again to Lord Vishnu for guidance. Lord Vishnu stepped up and brought Garuda, the divine bird, to help. Garuda lifted up the mountain easily as if it were a feather. Flapping his powerful wings, he took it over to the Kshirasagara and dropped it in the middle of the ocean. The Devatas then approached Vasuki, the king of serpents, and requested him to function as the rope. Vasuki agreed, so the Devatas and the Asuras wound the immense snake around the mountain and started churning.

However, having nothing to hold it at the base, the colossal mountain started sinking into the ocean. Lord Vishnu then assumed the avatar of Kurma and appeared as a heavenly tortoise. He swam under the mountain and held it on his back. Once again, the Devatas and the Asuras resumed churning, but this time, the mountain started slipping upwards. Now, Lord Vishnu assumed the avatar called Ajitha and appeared in a humanoid form to hold the Mandara Parvata down. Thus, supported by Lord Vishnu from above and from below, the mountain was finally held steady. The Devatas and the Asuras churned eagerly, drawing the serpent Vasuki back and forth. The waves grew higher and higher, cresting to unimaginable heights as the churning continued. And then, the Kshirasagara started responding and yielding all the wondrous and terrible things that lay in its depths.

First came Kaalakuta, the terrible poison that destroyed everything it touched. It roared through the realm, engulfing everything in its ruinous folds. Again, Lord Vishnu came to the rescue. He directed the foremost among the celestials, Mukhya Prana to swallow the poison, who immediately rescued all living things by swallowing the toxic poison entirely. While doing so, a few drops were also swallowed by Lord Shiva. When doing so, these drops of posion settled in Lord Shiva's throat. His throat took on a terrible blue tinge - and from that day on, Lord Shiva came to be known as Nilakantha - the blue-throated one.

The Kshirasagara then started giving up all its treasures. It yielded Airavata, the white elephant with four tusks. It gave up Uchchaisravas, a celestial horse, the first of its kind to be seen in this realm. It yielded Kamadhenu, the heavenly cow who grants anything one's heart desires. It birthed Lakshmi Devi, the Goddess of fortune, who was hence termed Jalaja, which means "one who is born of water." And then, out of Kshirasagara rose a resplendent being called Dhanvantari (who was none other than Lord Vishnu himself), carrying the pot of amrita in his arms. Amrita was the nectar of immortality—so as its bearer, Dhanvantari came to be known as the original physician and the preceptor of Ayurveda, which is the science/knowledge of life.

Ayurveda Then and Now

Today, a walk down any supermarket aisle will tell you how popular herbal cures have become. A quick browse online will tell you how going natural and organic is a whole lifestyle now. Of course, some of these changes are positive and extremely welcome in today's world. But there's also a lot of misinformation out there—many of which we'll explore in deeper detail in this book.

But the one thing that amuses me the most right now is when I see these concepts being marketed as something new! That's when I think back to that day when I first heard the story of the Samudra Manthana. I had always known that Ayurvedic knowledge and practices were an important part of my family's heritage, but until that day, I had no idea that the history went so long back.

Now, you might think that was just a tale told by a grandmother to her grandkids on a long-ago summer day. But most legends have a core of truth, and this one is no different. As I grew up and earned a PhD from the University of Utah in Biological Chemistry and then went on to do postdoctoral research at Stanford, I started doing my own research on Ayurveda. I was surprised to see that there were reliable mentions of medicine and medical practices in ancient Indian texts like the Vedas, Brahmanas, Aranyakas, and Upanishads. Some of these texts go back several millennia—and the medical practices described in these texts are considered revolutionary, even today.

Ancient Medicine—A Historical Throwback

Of course, there was a time when medicine was a magico-religious practice, with ailments being thought to be caused by divine imbalance, and priests playing the role of practitioners in society. But some of these beliefs went on to pave the way for a more practical school of thought. For instance, the juice of the soma plant was once thought to have the ability to make one immortal. But this brought people's attention to the fact that other plants may have curative properties too—and the ancient texts and legends show that plants and herbs were indeed used to cure illnesses. The *Rig Veda*, for instance, claims that "for a knowledgeable healer, the herbs rally together akin to an army of kings."

Folklore confirms this too. As one tale goes[1], a guruji in a gurukul once had three pupils. After he taught them all that he could, he set them a small challenge to test their knowledge. He gave them a month to travel, and during this time, they were to look for as many plants

---

1 Jivaka's story https://www.buddhistdoor.net/features/the-story-of-jivaka-the-buddhas-personal-physician

as they could find that did not have any useful properties. The three pupils took their leave and set out on their journey. At the end of the month, the first pupil brought back 50 different plants and lay them at the guruji's feet. The second pupil brought back 75. The third pupil, who was called Jivaka, came back empty-handed. 'What happened?' their guruji asked. 'Your peers covered a 50-kilometer radius from the gurukul and came back with so many plants. Did you not travel far enough?'

'On the contrary, I covered a 100-kilometer radius,' said Jivaka. 'But I couldn't see a single plant that I did not find any use for.' Their guruji finally cracked a smile. 'Bravo!' he said. 'You are the only scholar who seems to have paid attention to my teachings! Nature has provided us with a treasure trove of wealth in the form of plants and herbs. Each one has a unique value; you just have to know how to make use of it.'

The Birth of Ayurveda as a Codified System

Towards the later Vedic period, between 1000–600 BCE, medicine had started shifting away from magico-religious beliefs and was getting more rational and scientific. The *Atharva Veda* records detailed knowledge of human bones and other internal organs. It recognizes the role germs, worms, contaminated food, and unhealthy lifestyles play in causing various diseases. It differentiates between diseases and symptoms. Fever, for example, is not a disease in itself but is merely a symptom caused by some other illness. We know this today—and so did the doctors (or vaidyas as they were known) and priests thousands of years ago! The *Atharva Veda* even records the ancient understanding of hereditary diseases.

By 600 BCE, these ideas had become more methodically consolidated into the system we know today as Ayurveda. The major medical texts of the period, *Charaka Samhita* and *Sushruta Samhita,* set out logistical observations about various diseases in great detail. They refined the art of diagnostics and described multiple medical procedures in great detail. Moreover, this is also when medicine started being practiced by specially trained practitioners called vaidyas, rather than being a priest's secondary responsibility. These vaidyas were educated over several years, and just like our doctors today, they were given both theoretical and practical training before they could start treating patients. What's more, there are records of conferences and symposiums, where vaidyas would get together to exchange ideas and standardize Ayurvedic methods.

So, one can argue (and I vehemently do!) that nothing about Ayurveda is 'new-fangled' or 'alternative.' Western medicine has become popular only over the last 150–200 years—before that, plant-based and naturally derived Ayurvedic cures have been successfully used to treat people in India for thousands of years. Even today, a large majority of people in non-urban areas of India rely solely on Ayurveda as their only form of treatment. In many households across the country, herbal and plant-based cures are still a go-to solution for small malaises—grandmothers still offer honey, turmeric, and black pepper to their grandkids for sore throats. And to think the 'Turmeric Latte' has been trending for just a couple of years!

Vishakanyas and the Importance of Vaccines
Another idea that has grown to unhealthy proportions in recent years is the sudden and unwarranted suspicion of vaccines! Those who are against vaccination will have you believe that vaccines are a new concept thought up by pharmaceutical companies to make big bucks out of unsuspecting parents. But a little research into Ayurvedic concepts will reveal that the practice of vaccination and inoculation goes back thousands of years. They are, in fact, an important part of this medical system.

For thousands of years, Ayurvedic practitioners have understood the importance of immunizing oneself from various diseases. They were familiar with Swarna Prashana, which is the Ayurvedic method of immunizing a child, right from the time they are born. In fact, legend has it that ancient kings and courtesans even sought to build immunity to various poisons. Take the Vishakanyas for instance. As the term suggests, Vishakanyas were extremely venomous ladies ('Visha' translates to poison, and 'Kanya' refers to a young woman). They were said to have been female agents or assassins who were used as human weapons by kings. These female operatives would be sent to an enemy king's court as seductresses or courtiers. So toxic were these women, that a single drop of their bodily fluid—or as some texts suggest, even just their touch or breath—was enough to kill a human being. Some Sanskrit sources claim that one such Vishakanya was sent to assassinate Chandragupta Maurya, the first emperor of the Maurya dynasty. The Vishakanya is mentioned in the *Arthashastra*, which is a treatise on governance written by Chandragupta Maurya's advisor, Chanakya.

Now, a woman who can ooze poison and kill on touch may sound like a stretch, but this legend is actually derived from the concept of 'Oka Satmya.' This refers to the practice of building up immunity to certain substances gradually, through long-time exposure and adaptation. Vishakanyas were said to have been administered minute doses of various snake venoms and poisons from the time they were born. Through the years, these women developed an almost superhuman immunity to all kinds of venoms and toxins. The idea being that they could infiltrate an enemy king's court, serve poisoned food or wine to the king, and gain their trust by drinking from the same plate or goblet without being affected by the poison themselves. And not just Vishakanyas—many kings themselves were said to have been immunized against poisons in a similar way to ward off attacks and attempts on their lives. In the West, this practice is known as Mithridatism.

Again, though such tales may seem like, well, just tales, the concepts they are rooted in have huge relevance in our lives today. Of course, given that enemies with murderous intent are not such a huge problem for most of us in our everyday lives (I hope!), we can probably skip building tolerance to poisons. However, building immunity and preventing diseases is something we all realize the importance of, especially right now, as the world comes to a screeching halt with the COVID-19 pandemic.

The world today is pretty flat. COVID-19 originated in Wuhan (China) in December 2019 (maybe even earlier, who knows!). Within weeks, the virus had spread to different corners of the world. With international travel being an important part of our lifestyle now, we cannot rest assured that a disease that has broken out in one part of the globe will not be at our doorstep tomorrow. Nor can we hope to predict the way different disease-causing microorganisms will mutate. So, the best course of action right now is to vaccinate ourselves against the most common diseases and then focus on building non-specific immunity. This cannot be achieved by popping pills to treat symptoms or tackling diseases as they come up. And that's exactly where Ayurveda comes in.

With that, let us delve into the different concepts and practices of Ayurveda, explore how they can help us in our daily lives today—and also debunk some myths while we are at it.

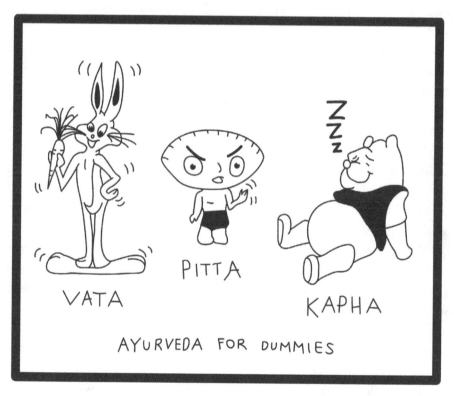

VATA

PITTA

KAPHA

AYURVEDA FOR DUMMIES

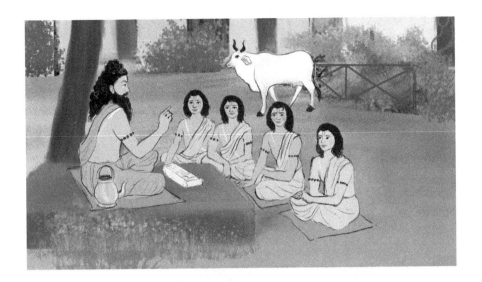

CHAPTER 2

Sushruta and the Nose Job: Heroes of Ayurveda

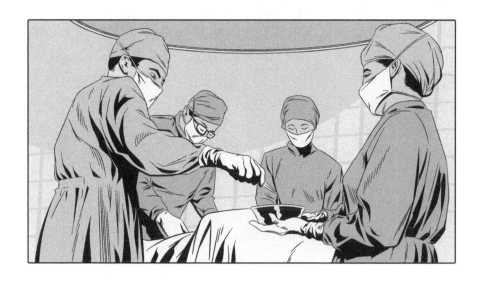

IT WAS A Saturday evening—one of the rare ones when I was done with work early and had the rest of the day to myself. I was pretty excited because an old college buddy was in town, and we had planned to catch up after work. Venu and I had been inseparable back in the day, and even moving countries, moving jobs, and going through big life changes had not been enough to make us lose touch. I was looking forward to an evening of coffee and reminiscences—after all, no one but a college mate will remember the particular pain of being confronted with sloppy hostel food on a day when you have a big paper due!

I was also eager to see Venu because I knew he had been going through some health issues of late. He hadn't gone into much detail over the phone, but he had mentioned it was something to do with his heart. Knowing him as I do, I could tell that he was trying to mask how worried he actually was. In fact, the reason he was in town was that he had an appointment with a heart specialist earlier that day.

I stepped into the café and spotted Venu right away. He was sitting at a corner table, a steaming cup of coffee in front of him. He didn't look remotely worried or tense—if anything, he looked . . . relaxed! I went over to join him. After a few exciting minutes of catching up, and a few more spent perusing the menu (a far cry from hostel food!), I asked him about his health scare. 'You had me worried when we spoke on the phone earlier. What happened?'

'It was a couple of weeks ago. I was in a meeting and I started having these sharp pains in my chest,' Venu said. 'I thought I'd better get it checked, so I left work early and went to the most famous hospital in town. After listening to my issue, they referred me to a heart specialist—he is the best, they said. The doctor asked me a couple of questions, and then said the pain could be due to a variety of reasons.'

'Did he zero in on a reason?' I enquired.

'Well, no. He said at my age, it could be anything—and that he needed to run some tests to be sure. What followed was two weeks of running back and forth from the hospital, getting the tests done, waiting for the results, going in for follow-ups, being told the results were inconclusive, being sent for more tests . . . you know how it is. I tried to keep calm, but by the end of the second week, I was close to losing it! That's why, when someone referred this specialist in Chennai, I flew in right away.' At this point, for some inexplicable reason, Venu started looking kind of sheepish.

'And? What did the specialist say it was?' I asked.

'Gas.'

The Lost Art of Diagnostics

I'm glad that Venu's story was something we could (and did, uproariously) laugh about. But this got me thinking about the lost art of diagnostics. If you live in an urban center in India and you feel unwell, chances are you'd take exactly the same course of action that Venu did. You would call a nearby hospital to make an appointment. The receptionist would ask you what your issue is and then go ahead and book you a slot with a specialist doctor in that field. Or perhaps you'd already have a name in mind—a specialist your friend recommended—and you'd request an appointment with that doctor.

But as we are slowly coming to realize, reaching out to a specialist right from the get-go is not the perfect solution. Here's why:

1. When you choose your specialist, you are making your choice based on the symptoms you notice. And if you're not a doctor yourself, you may not be reading the symptoms correctly. As in Venu's case, his chest pain was caused by something that he, as a non-medical professional, would never have connected.

2. The other issue with the modern system we follow . . . even if you happen to read your symptoms correctly and choose the right specialist, you are more likely to be getting a cookie-cutter solution. The specialist will send you for some tests, examine the results, and suggest a line of treatment based on what they see on that one piece of paper. This is known as evidence-based medicine—a system where the treatment is influenced by test results alone. Now, this system has its pros, but it also has some gaping flaws—the main one being that the diagnosis you get is not personalized to your particulars. Let me give you a very simplistic example. Say you are a woman in her 20s–30s and are experiencing unexplained hair fall, so the specialist sends you for a complete blood count (CBC) test. The results of that test show that your hemoglobin levels are low. Now, anybody who exhibits low levels of hemoglobin

will be given the same medicines and treatment. But unexplained hair fall can be due to low hemoglobin levels (in fact, anemia is indeed the number one cause for hair fall in women in India as well as other parts of the world, which explains why your doctor sent you in for this test in particular), as well as a poorly functioning liver. But the specialist, not knowing your particular history, doesn't know which one it is—so they are most likely to give you a drug to bring the hemoglobin levels up and may still not solve the problem. So, it is paramount that your doctor actually spends time with you, speaks to you, understands your lifestyle, and THEN comes up with an intelligent diagnosis. Evidence-based medicine is both a boon and a bane.

However, a physician who takes the time to learn the specifics about your lifestyle and family history and asks you the right questions is more likely to diagnose you correctly. Sometime not so long ago, most of us had 'family doctors'—trusted general physicians (GPs) whom we would reach out to whenever anybody in the family fell ill. These were typically long-term engagements, where these doctors would know you at a personal level. They would be familiar with your lifestyle, your medical history, and, having treated your parents and maybe even grandparents, they'd know about any underlying genetic conditions too. Being privy to so much background information, they'd easily be able to differentiate the smaller issues and treat them right at their clinic. Of course, they might have prescribed certain tests to confirm their diagnosis. But they would at least have known the direction in which to proceed, rather than just sending you in for every test under the sun, hoping to get a hit somewhere. For more serious issues, they'd tell you which specialist to consult, and perhaps even refer you to someone they know to be good. With the popularity of multi-specialty hospitals today, these independent general practices are on the ebb. If Venu had a trusted GP he could have turned to, it might have saved him a lot of stress and of course, thousands in medical bills.

The Egg White-Avocado Conundrum

Even a decade or so back, egg yolks were a big no-no. Doctors would warn you against them. Nutritionists would suggest alternatives. Buff actors talking about their diets would tell you about how many egg whites they had per day—but not the yolk, never the yolk! The reason? They were thought to be extremely dense in cholesterol. And of course, cholesterol is *bad*!

Now cut to the present. The egg yolk is back in business. Avocados are trending. Red wine is good for you. So what happened to all those high cholesterol scares? Here's the thing—medical research is always evolving. Every year, we learn new things that we didn't know the year before. Today, we know that there are good and bad kinds of cholesterols. While the bad kind might clog your arteries and give you heart trouble, the good kind will actually help keep said arteries healthy.

So you missed out on some good meals that you could have enjoyed—but other than that, no harm was done, right? Now here comes the tricky bit. Back when doctors still thought all cholesterols were bad, a whole lot of people were prescribed these cholesterol-lowering drugs called statins. And what's the problem with statins?

Back in my graduate college days, when I was studying in the U.S., I was aghast to see the advertisements they had for different brands of medicines. These ads would talk about what the medicine does, and then prompt you to ask your doctor to prescribe that drug for you if you're having those symptoms. (Call me old-fashioned, but I think it's the doctor who should do the prescribing!) But what amused me the most was that these ads would always end with a long list of side effects—and some of the side effects were exactly what the drug was supposed to prevent in the first place! And that is the issue with statins, in a nutshell.

New research has shown that these cholesterol-lowering drugs have a list of side effects as long as my arm. Milder fallouts include nausea, dizziness, and muscle weakness. More severe side effects extend to damaged kidneys and (you guessed it) heart problems—the one thing it was supposed to prevent. And the kicker is that you don't want to get rid of all types of cholesterol after all. And why is that—because cholesterol is necessary to build the structure of cell membranes, make hormones like estrogen, testosterone and adrenal hormones, essential for your body to produce vitamin D. That apart, cholesterol is essential to produce bile acids, which help the body digest fat and absorb important nutrients. Do you see the irony here? You need cholesterol to help digest fat!

If you have 'high cholesterol,' making changes in your diet can help bring it down into the healthy range. Exercise can help boost the level of protective high-density lipoproteins (HDL) and prevent your body from producing more cholesterol. Statins should NEVER be the go-to solution for lowering levels of low-density lipoproteins (LDL)—at least in my considered opinion.

Diagnostics the Ayurvedic Way

The one thing you should know about Ayurveda is that it is a very holistic practice. Its main aim is to prevent and relieve illness and improve one's quality of life. The word 'Ayurveda' literally means the science/knowledge of life. It doesn't just focus on the disease or symptoms in isolation—it also looks at the person as a whole. So, if you go in with a headache, that's unlikely to be the only thing Ayurveda will treat, nor will the practitioner give you a pill to pop, which he gives all other patients with headaches. Ayurveda establishes the whys, the whens, and the hows. It'll find out why you are suffering from a headache. Is it genetic? Is it a fallout of your lifestyle? Were you exposed to certain elements that did not agree with your unique constitution? Answering all these questions and more is what Ayurvedic diagnosis is all about.

A visit to an Ayurvedic practitioner would be no five-minute appointment. The practitioner will spend at least half an hour asking you various questions. In fact, if you are not familiar with Ayurvedic methods, you might be quite taken aback at the detailed interrogation! After all, most people are not used to their doctors enquiring about their mental capacity, what a typical day at work looks like, and specifics about the kind of foods they eat. But interrogation or 'prashna' is an important part of

Ayurvedic diagnosis—the third step in a comprehensive 12-step process known as dvadashavidha pariksha (or 12-step diagnosis)Apart from these questions, an Ayurvedic practitioner will also put their power of observation (darshana) to use, making careful note of your complexion, the color of your eyes, the state of your nails, lips, and so on. They will carry out sparshana—a physical inspection through touch, where they may feel your pulse, press your stomach, and tap your joints. This is well elaborated in a treatise called Charaka Samhita (Vimanasthana, Chapter 1, verse 3), which every keen student of Ayurveda must be well-versed with or at least have a more-than-passing familiarity with. To very briefly describe this process, the physician must first comprehend the features of the disease in terms of etiology, prodroma (period between the time of first appearance of symptoms to the full-blown presentation of the condition), symptoms, suitability of the treatment, number of medicines to be given, predominance of the symptoms, types of symptoms, proportional variation, severity and time. He then needs to carefully analyze and understand the features of the doshas (a purely Ayurvedic term that really has no equivalent word in the English language. Loosely, it can be translated to meaning the forces— for lack of a better term—that constitute the physical body), drugs, place, time, strength, body type, diet, psyche, constitution of the individual, age, and suitability of the body for a particular treatment. Through an extensive process of observation, experimentation, and inference, they will collate enough information to be able to diagnose your illness, ascertain why it has occurred, and advise you about the best way to treat it.

So, who established this detailed method of diagnosis?

Ancient Pioneers: Three Heroes of Ayurveda

On August 20, 1897, Surgeon-Major Ronald Ross made a landmark discovery. He proved that malaria parasites are transmitted to humans through mosquitos—the anopheles mosquito, to be more specific. Malaria is one disease that has plagued the human race for thousands of years. There are references to the disease in Mesopotamian clay tablets, Homer's writings, and ancient Chinese and Roman accounts. But before this discovery by Ross, nobody had any clear idea of how exactly this disease was transmitted.

Of course, many people tried to note the commonalities and make educated guesses. Some ancient scholars believed that it only occurred in low-lying, tropical areas. But that wasn't quite true, as cases of malaria were noted in temperate areas too, while some tropical areas seemed to be safe from the disease. Other scholars and medical professionals did make the connection with marshy, swampy, or waterlogged areas. But they thought it was the fumes or evil vapors emitted by marshes that caused the disease. In fact, the term 'malaria' actually comes from the Italian *mal'aria*, which means 'bad air.' Eventually, it was in 1880 that a French doctor named Alphonse Laveran discovered the malaria parasite. And some years after that, Ross linked the transmission to mosquito bites—a discovery considered to be one of the greatest medical breakthroughs of our times.

Now, let's go back a couple of thousand years, to the seventh or sixth century BCE. A physician in ancient India sits writing in his journal. He looks through a list—a list of hundreds of insects, worms, germs, and animals that he has observed to cause diseases in human beings. In the end, he adds five more items to the list—five different kinds of mosquitos!

1. Sushruta

This physician was Sushruta. His compendium, the *Sushruta Samhita,* remains one of the greatest treatises of ancient Ayurvedic medicine. Not much is known about the person himself, except that he practiced medicine in the northern part of India that today is known as Varanasi. The other thing we know is that he lived in the seventh or sixth century BCE. This puts him at a time much before the birth of the Greek physician Hippocrates, who came to be known as the 'Father of Medicine.'

The *Sushruta Samhita* was written as a guidebook or an instruction manual for later physicians. It is startling for its detailed descriptions of various medical procedures and its precise, step-by-step instructions for surgical techniques, all peppered with Sushruta's own comments and practical observations. He writes about more than a thousand ailments and diseases and proceeds to talk about the treatments for these. He mentions over 700 medicinal herbs that can be used for various kinds of cures.

The number of surgical procedures he talks about runs into hundreds, with over 120 different kinds of instruments. Surgery was practiced even before Sushruta's time, but the way he refined the existing techniques was astounding. One interesting innovation is his method for suturing internal surgical wounds. He used black ants, which bit down on both sides of the wound, clamping it shut. Then, the physician removed the body of the ants, keeping the ant heads in place. Once the wound had healed enough, the ant heads would be absorbed by the body—an important point, given that we're talking internal surgery here. Sushruta also paved the way for alcohol and cannabis-based anesthetics—he used alcohol to render a patient insensible before they underwent surgery.

Now, what can this genius who lived thousands of years ago possibly have in common with a modern Hollywood/Bollywood starlet? The title of this chapter gives you a hint!

Indeed, no discussion about Sushruta would be complete without a mention of one of his most noteworthy contributions—his innovations in the field of cosmetic surgery. Rhinoplasty (or the nose job) was his specialty, and he developed the technique of nose reconstructive surgery to a great extent. Of course, in Sushruta's time, a 'nose job' had deeper implications than it does today. One of the most common forms of punishment back then was rhinotomy, which is when one's nose is cut off. Rhinotomy was used to mark out criminals, as well as punish and shame women suspected of adultery. Suspected, not even convicted, mind you! Of course, once one had their nose cut off, stigma and disgrace would follow them wherever they went. Sushruta and his reconstructive rhinoplasty gave countless people a second lease of life—and the good doctor left detailed notes so that thousands of years later, we know the exact process he followed.

Coming back to Ayurvedic diagnosis, that's another thing that Sushruta focused on. In his lifetime, he took on several students (who were referred to as the Saushrutas) whom he passed his knowledge on to. His course was as intensive as anything our doctors go through today. Just like our modern practices, his students started off by taking an oath. They then went on to train under Sushruta for six years, during which time he taught them how to identify, diagnose, treat and cure diseases.

The course involved dissection and analysis of corpses in order to understand the internal organs and the skeletal structure. This is something that physicians in Europe couldn't do for a long time, given their prohibitions on corpse dissection. In the course of their training, the students first practiced their surgical knowledge on softwood, vegetation, and animal remains. Only once they mastered these did they 'graduate' to more hands-on surgeries.

Moving away from specializations, Sushruta insisted that a physician should know every aspect of the body's functioning to be able to treat and prevent diseases effectively. This included knowing about the causes and effects of environmental factors, genetic markers, and lifestyle. He encouraged his students to carry out detailed questions so that they were able to come to the root of the issue. His methods enabled him and his students to make the art of healing more scientific, without resorting to amulets or supernatural explanations.

2. Charaka
Remember how we talked about the scholars who tried to connect outbreaks of malaria with lowlands or marshes? There was another ancient Indian physician who was an expert at the concept of medical geography. This physician was called Acharya Charaka, who is also known as the 'Father of Indian Medicine.' He lived and worked during the second century BC (this is as per a calculation based on various references to *Charaka Samhita*. The exact date of his birth and death are not well-documented). He is believed to have been the royal physician of King Kanishka.

Several centuries before Charaka, there was a great sage by the name of Punarvasu Atreya, who had developed and written about many Ayurvedic concepts in depth. Atreya had six disciples, all of whom produced a compendium (or samhita) where they wrote down Atreya's teachings along with their own thoughts. Of these disciples' work, the treatise by Agnivesha was found to be the most comprehensive and well organized. Centuries later, Charaka refined, developed, and annotated Agnivesha's ideas, thereby creating a brand-new compendium that came to be known as *Charaka Samhita*. Along with the *Sushruta Samhita* and *Ashtanga Hridayam*, the *Charaka Samhita* makes up the 'Big Three' of the ancient Ayurvedic texts.

The *Charaka Samhita* makes a comprehensive correlation between geographical factors in the diagnosis and treatment of diseases. For instance, when talking about epidemics, he expounds his theories on the Gangetic plains. Likewise, he also identifies the different pharmaceutical plants that are available in different regions. Indeed, many curative plants and drugs are named after the region they come from. Charaka also notes how the people of certain communities may have developed specific tolerances based on the dietary habits typical of their geographical region.

Whereas Sushruta attained fame for his contributions in the surgical field, Charaka is renowned for his work in the branch of medicine known as 'Kayachikitsa,' which mainly deals with diagnosis and treatment of various general health problems. He was the first physician to expound theories about metabolism, digestion, and immunity. He observed the effects of different kinds of food on the body and believed that diseases were caused by unwholesome diets. Earlier, the concept of predetermination of life was prevalent—people believed that one's lifespan was already decided by higher powers and could not be altered, no matter what one did. But Charaka was strongly opposed to this. He proposed that a healthy, wholesome lifestyle coupled with good nutrition could prevent diseases and prolong one's life. Preventive medical practices were given a high degree of importance by this Acharya—in fact, he placed them higher than the treatment. (Prevention is better than cure—sound familiar?)

Today, the concept of healthy living seems to have become confused with extreme austerity and self-denial. People cut out fat, carbs, sugar, and other 'unhealthy' things mercilessly from their diets, believing they are making a positive change. Some people eat only fruits; others feel extremely guilty if they so much as touch a dessert. This sometimes tends to be even more counterintuitive than the occasional junk meal. At least, when you are having junk food, you are under no illusions—you know it's unhealthy and that you should probably not have all those fried snacks too regularly. But when people think that they are actually making a healthy choice by cutting out a food group completely, they are more likely to keep it up longer. And if they happen to make these changes without any expert guidance, they may end up doing lasting damage to their body.

If these people had consulted Charaka, they may have been a lot happier, for he promoted moderation in all things. He believed that health does not just pertain to physical wellness. One has to be happy and fulfilled in order to be truly healthy—and constant abstinence and asceticism are no way to achieve that! His compendium recommends a moderate, well-balanced diet that features a bit of everything, including meats, fats, alcohol, and the smoking of medicinal herbs. However, he sets out meticulous guidelines for the consumption of such items—the correct quantities, the right time to consume them, and the safe food combinations to consume them with. Again, he was very clear that not everyone was allowed to eat all these. There were particular conditions in which he advocated each of the above. He also notes the fallouts of overindulgence. Moreover, he sets out recommendations for tailoring one's diets with the changing seasons. What's more, Charaka was instrumental in systematizing medical diagnoses, and he developed a scientific method of diagnosis. He was also the first to put forth the approach of the psychosomatic origin of diseases. He was the first to come up with an individualized treatment regimen for any disease. Like we discussed earlier, one size does NOT fit all. We owe that methodology to Charaka—and how right he was!

3. Jivaka

Now let's meet the third pioneer of ancient Ayurveda—a physician called Jivaka. Jivaka lived in the fifth century BC and was Buddha's personal physician. It is said that Jivaka was born to a courtesan, who left him for dead in a rubbish heap. Bimbisara was the king of Magadha at the time, and his son, Prince Abhaya, happened to be out on a stroll on that particular day. Prince Abhaya came across the newborn child in the rubbish heap and adopted him as his son. The name 'Jivaka' is derived from the Pali words meaning 'one who lived.'

Jivaka grew up with a thirst for knowledge and an interest in medicine. He trained under a renowned physician in Takshashila. His understanding of the curative properties of plants and herbs was astonishing. (He is said to have been the disciple we spoke of in the previous chapter—the one who failed to find a single useless plant for his guruji.) One of the first instances of Jivaka's proficiency was when he was on his way back home after his medical training was complete. As the story goes, Jivaka ran out of money halfway through his journey. To raise enough funds, he went around the town he was in, offering his services as a physician to anyone who needed it. Although initially hesitant, a wealthy merchant's wife enlisted his help. She had been suffering from terrible headaches for many years, and no other practitioner had been able to cure her so far. After carrying out the 'dvadashividha pariksha' or the 12-fold method of patient examination, Jivaka diagnosed her correctly. He was able to offer the right cure—a preparation made from ghee and herbs, to be taken nasally. The happy patient's family rewarded Jivaka with gold coins, a horse, and other riches.

Once home, Jivaka became King Bimbisara's physician. He also treated other kings of allied kingdoms, earning great wealth along the way. In the meantime, King Bimbisara had embraced the tenets of Buddhism and had become Buddha's host and sponsor. As the royal physician, Jivaka also started treating Buddha and his monks. Jivaka understood the importance of a clean environment and good personal hygiene. As per the monastic rules back then, monks were required to wear robes pieced together from discarded rags collected at cemeteries. Jivaka correlated this practice with multiple diseases. He is said to have talked Buddha into moving away from this rule and allowing his monks to accept donated garments instead.

The Vaidya

Over the centuries, these physicians and scholars shaped the Ayurvedic practice as we know it today. Among their teachings, they also set out guidelines for how vaidyas or Ayurvedic practitioners should comport themselves. According to Sushruta, a vaidya should not only be intelligent and scholarly but should also have the ability to apply their acquired knowledge in practical situations. Vaidyas had to be patient, well spoken, and observant. Just like any doctor today, vaidyas were licensed by the state and had to live up to certain standards in their practice. Both Sushruta and Charaka expressed strong opinions against charlatans and quacks and called for them to be set distinctly apart from legitimate vaidyas.

As we discussed earlier in the chapter, specializations were unheard of—a vaidya was expected to have a thorough understanding of the entire human body and be proficient in all the different branches of medicine. Their training was supposed to cover not just knowledge about the therapeutic properties of plants and herbs, but also their side effects. They were supposed to weigh the pros and cons of a particular line of treatment before recommending it to a patient. Had statins existed back then, no vaidya would have come within ten miles of it!

To this day, Ayurvedic practitioners are trained to know the side effects of anything they prescribe. For example, if you went to a vaidya with symptoms of a heart problem, and after preliminary examination, it is indeed found to be a heart-related issue, the vaidya would prescribe a decoction made from Arjuna bark, mainly because Arjuna possesses anti-ischemic, antioxidant, hypolipidemic (reduces LDL levels), and antiatherogenic (prevents the formation of plaques) activities. Of course, one should procure these decoctions or kashayams or kadhas from a bona fide, regulatory-compliant, government-approved pharmacy, which carries such formulations and medicines from authentic manufacturers. As far as Ayurveda goes, a cure that causes more harm than good is considered to be no cure at all.

Chapter 3

Heavy, Heavy Fuel: Myths Associated with Raw Materials, Metals, and Minerals

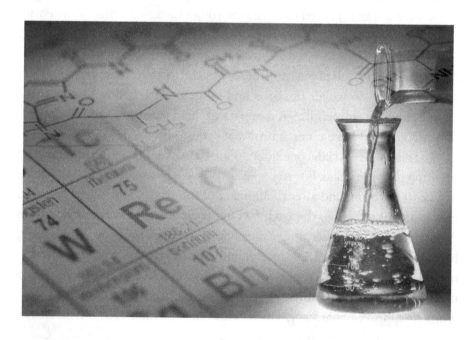

A MID-SPRING MORNING long ago, my brother and I are awoken at an unearthly hour and hurried off to the bathroom to bathe and get ready in our new clothes. Still rubbing sleep from my eyes, I stumble behind my mother, who's carrying my brother in her arms. It is Rama Navami, and after bathing and getting dressed, I am to help my parents and grandparents prepare for the puja that day.

The sun is pretty low in the sky, so the morning is still quite cool. Of course, later in the day, it would be sizzling hot in typical Chennai fashion. But for now, the ground is cool below my bare feet, and I shiver as a mug of cold water is poured on my head. But though I am tired and sleepy and cold, I don't mind any of it one bit. You see, there is something that's driving me ahead—something I am looking forward to very much.

I must have been about seven then—too young to know much about why certain festivals are celebrated. I did not yet know about their implications or the importance they held for my family. The one thing I did know though was that after the puja was over, I would get to sit down to one of my grandmother's feasts.

This feast was not designed to just appeal to the tastebuds—it was a feast for your eyes and nose too. Imagine a heavy silver plate. At the center, there would be a perfect mound of the most fragrant puliogare—tamarind rice seasoned with spices, herbs, and seeds. The choicest traditional delicacies would sit all around it. A helping of kosambari, a cold salad made of soaked mung dal, shaved veggies, and raw mangoes from our trees. A serving of bisi bele bath, tempered with curry leaves and accompanied by appalam (papad). A bowl of black gram prepared with herbs and grated coconut. And of course, the sweet treats—gulab jamuns, payasam (rice pudding), and coconut laddoos. On the side, there would be two copper glasses. One would be filled with spiced buttermilk (unfortunately I am allergic to buttermilk, but I hear that it's amazing); the other with panakam—a cool drink made with jaggery, lemon, ginger, and other spices (I would always request a second helping of this one). Tell me you wouldn't wake up early for a feast like that!

The Wisdom of a Grandmother's Kitchen

Of course, my memories of my grandmother's kitchen go much beyond the feasts. I still think about the massive tins of laddoos that she would prepare and keep. The endless jars of various kinds of pickles that she would bring out with a flourish during mealtimes. Even the way her kitchen looked was very different from any kitchen I see today. The burnished red oxide floor. The walls and shelves stacked with scrubbed matte pots and pans, made of bell metal and brass. The massive kadhais made of cast iron and clay. On one side, there was a round-bottomed copper jar that stored drinking water and kept it naturally cool in the balmy Chennai summers.

Kids today, of course, will have very different memories when they grow up. They'll remember our modular kitchens, our aluminum utensils, and our plastic storage containers. Indeed, as we graduated to our more modern kitchens, we opted out of the culinary lifestyle of our grandparents' generation. Rather than the matte bronzes and bell metals, we have our gleaming stainless steel. Rather than maintaining and tempering a cast-iron skillet, we prefer our Teflon-coated non-stick pans. Not all of it is just for the sake of convenience either—after all, storing water in a copper vessel is no more trouble than storing it in a plastic bottle. Perhaps then, it is the aesthetic preferences that have changed.

However, there's one little thing that we missed factoring in—our grandparents were not using metal and earthen vessels for their rustic aesthetics. Nor were they indulging in a spot of nostalgia. These practices actually had some tangible value. Today, many of us take a wide array of vitamin and mineral supplements to stay healthy and fit. In some countries, you can even have vitamin subscriptions—where you just fill out a questionnaire and the right supplements are shipped home every month. But back when there was no easy access to pill supplements, these practices were carried out in a more everyday way—like a grandma cooking in a copper or clay pot.

When you cook and store food in certain kinds of vessels, microparticles and minerals and nanodoses of metals from those vessels are infused naturally into your food and go into your system as a part of your daily meals. The quantity of metals you ingest this way is very small—not enough to cause you any harm and not even enough to alter the taste of food in any significant way. But it is just enough to ensure that you get your supplements in, safely and regularly.

The War Against 'Chemicals'

Now, if someone tells you your utensils are leaching metals into your food, your first reaction might be to get alarmed. You might take it as an indication that the vessels were not well made, and immediately start worrying about the health implications for your family. Indeed, it is a smart move to invest in good quality kitchenware, but don't ask for your money back just yet. Here's why—leaching metals in itself is not so alarming if it's the right kind and quantity of metals.

So why do we get alarmed when we hear something like this? The top reason I can think of is because of the modern suspicion of chemicals. In the first chapter, I talked about the new wave of natural living that has become popular. While I reiterate that living a simpler and more organic lifestyle can be a great thing, I strongly believe in the importance of making such lifestyle changes in a practical, educated way. All too often, I see people wholeheartedly embracing anything that says 'natural' on the label, without any further questions. And on the flip side of the coin, they automatically suspect anything that they think is chemical. Seeing anything long, complicated, or vaguely 'chemical-sounding' in the list of ingredients will convince them that the product is bad!

See the problem? I can think of two issues with this right away:

1. Not everything that is natural is good for you (especially when improperly used). Certain kinds of plants and flowers are highly toxic. You know not to pick up and eat random berries or mushrooms while you're out hiking because some of them can kill you. Moreover, not everyone reacts to natural elements the same way. Even something as mundane as peanuts or shrimps can be fatal to those who are allergic to them.
2. Everything around us is made of chemicals. We tend to think of chemicals as something essentially new, artificial, and harmful—but that's of course not true. Even common, everyday natural items have their own unique chemical compositions. For example, you can safely consume 2-hydroxypropane-1,2,3-tricarboxylic acid

every day—that's just the citric acid in lemon juice. When some-one adds 8-methyl-N-vanillyl-6-nonenamideto your food, they're not trying to kill you—they're just seasoning your food with red chili powder.

So, whether or not something has chemicals is no indication of how good or bad it is. If you do not have a background in chemistry or medicine, a label may not tell you much. You may need to do further, in-depth research to truly understand the properties of those compounds. Likewise, just because metals and minerals feature on the periodic table we remember from our chemistry classes, it doesn't mean they're bad. Most of these occur naturally in the food we eat—and trace amounts are even found in our bodies.

Metals in Our Body

We need metals for the healthy functioning of various systems in our bodies. Most of us know this already, in a theoretical way—but chances are we don't give much thought to the practical implications of this. So, here's a quick roundup of some of the common metals and minerals we need, and the ways in which they help.

- **Iron**: It is needed for the proper functioning of our red blood cells—it is contained in hemoglobin, which carries oxygen to dif-ferent parts of our body. When you don't have enough iron in your body, you tend to become anemic.
- **Copper**: This helps the body produce red blood cells and enables us to metabolize fuels. It also regulates the absorption of iron and is an important component of many structural proteins in our body. Copper deficiency is marked by anemia, muscle weakness, and neurological disorders.
- **Zinc**: This makes up various proteins in our body. It is also extremely important for the proper functioning of our nervous and immune systems. Zinc is vital for the proper functioning of both the male and female reproductive systems. Zinc has also been

linked to the brain's capacity to learn new things and form memories. Zinc deficiency and imbalance compromise the immune system and have been associated with Alzheimer's disease.

- **Potassium**: Potassium balances and maintains the intracellular fluids in the body, and regulates blood pressure and heartbeats. If you experience weakness, fatigue, muscle cramps, and heart irregularities, potassium deficiency can be a potential cause. A vast majority (about 97 percent) of Americans have been noted to have this deficiency.[2]
- **Calcium**. As most of us already know, this helps build healthy bones and teeth. But calcium also has its uses in our nervous system as well as for proper muscle function. Not having enough calcium in the body can cause diseases like osteoporosis and osteopenia, which make bones brittle with a tendency to fracture easily.
- **Sodium**. It controls nerve impulses and regulates muscle functions. Having low levels of sodium in the body is called hyponatremia, and it can cause nausea, dizziness, confusion, and disorientation, with more severe cases even resulting in coma or death.

A healthy, balanced diet can help us get many of the minerals we need—but we might not be able to get the necessary levels of metals needed in our body through diet alone. These then, need to be added in. This can be done with pills and supplements. Or it can be made available to your body in more everyday ways—like cooking your food in cast iron or clay vessels.

Rasashaastra

So far, we have only discussed the benefits of plants and herbs in Ayurvedic treatments—but there's one field of Ayurvedic study that we haven't touched upon yet. This branch is called Rasashaastra, which refers to the study of the therapeutic properties of metals and minerals. The role that metals and minerals play in our bodies is well known to us today—and it was also known to our ancestors centuries ago.

---

2 https://www.ncbi.nlm.nih.gov/pmc/articles/PMC3650509/

Rasashaastra is an in-depth study of the properties and functions of 'Khanija' or 'Paarthiwa' materials—which basically refers to materials that are derived from mineral sources. Ancient physicians like Sushruta and Charaka were well aware of the therapeutic properties of minerals. *Charaka Samhita,* for instance, lists formulations made of different kinds of iron, gold, silver, copper, brass, bronze, and so on. Charaka recommended the use of some types of iron to treat anemia, inflammatory disorders, and eye and skin diseases. He noted the benefits of copper in the treatment of many respiratory diseases as well as eye and skin infections. He listed formulations of gold and silver for their rejuvenative properties and for the treatment of certain kinds of tumors, blood disorders, and fevers. Rasashaastra, however, was developed into a specialized field of study by the Buddhist sage, Naagaarjuna.

The Concept of Bioavailability

Whereas plants, herbs, and animal-based materials do not need much processing to be consumable, it was recognized that metals and minerals are not compatible with the human body in their natural forms. Rasashaastra, thus, also involved an understanding of how these substances could be processed to make them safe for human consumption.

Take anemia for instance—1.62 billion people around the world are affected by it, with iron deficiency being the most common cause for it. If you are diagnosed with this, you are going to have to find a way to restore the levels of iron in your body. Now, obviously, you will not just swallow some pieces of iron—and not least because that's going to be a tad uncomfortable! Common sense tells you that the iron is not in a form that's assimilable by your body.

Though this might be an overly simplistic example, the concept holds even when you are given the supplement in a pill. It's not just enough for the iron to enter your body, it has to be administered in a bioavailable form—a form that your body will be able to absorb easily. Unfortunately, that is a huge issue with many allopathic pill supplements out there. Given how common anemia is, especially among women, a whole lot of people are prescribed iron supplements. But the iron contained within is a synthesized, inorganic form of the metal that is not bioavailable. The result is that only a small portion of the given amount is managed to be absorbed by the body—with the rest getting deposited on various organs. As you may have probably guessed—not a good thing!. It can cause a plethora of side effects and complications including nausea, constipation, griping, and even kidney malfunction.

Ayurvedic technology, on the other hand, is extremely advanced when it comes to making materials bioavailable. Ayurvedic supplements of iron (or zinc or copper) are treated in a way that makes the metals more assimilable. So not only does it eliminate the risk of organ deposition and other side effects, but it also means that you need to take a far smaller quantity of it—since whatever little that is administered gets absorbed by the body, taking a large dose is not necessary. Ayurvedic technology also has the ability to ensure that a particular drug is delivered to the correct site within your body and to ensure that your immune system reacts optimally to it.

The technology that allows Ayurvedic practitioners to achieve this is the original form of nanomedicine. The metals or minerals are converted to a form called 'bhasma,' which is fine ash or powder. Bhasma is prepared by purifying the given substance, treating it with particular plant extracts or juices, and then incinerating it into a fine powder. There are specific guidelines for preparing Bhasmas out of different metals, keeping in mind their specific qualities. Properly incinerated bhasma has to meet certain set standards too—for instance, it has to be tasteless, lusterless, and has to float on water. Once it is prepared, the bhasma has to be mixed with a formulation of the right herbs and plant materials before it is consumed.

Even today, Ayurvedic technology remains far superior to allopathic techniques in many ways. Not only does this technology make the material more bioavailable, but it also makes it safer. Take sulfur for instance. A lot of allopathic medicines, ointments, and skin creams use sulfur for its therapeutic properties. Now, there are three forms of sulfur that can be used in medicinal formulations—sublimed, precipitated, or colloidal sulfur.

While colloidal sulfur is the preferred form because it has a diverse array of uses including dermatological and as internal antibiotic, the modern techniques used to make colloidal sulfur are low-yielding and very expensive. In Ayurveda, however, the usage of purified sulfur is de rigueur. There is a formulation called 'Rasagandhaka,' which is a preparation of sulfur and mercury, and that forms the basis of many Ayurvedic medications and treatments—both external and internal.

Heavy Metals

Did you notice the word mercury in the previous sentence? If you just got alarmed, I'll bet you're not alone. Indeed, in our living memory, mercury has come to be associated with something terribly toxic. The very term 'heavy metal' causes discomfort. After all, most of us have read about the Minamata disease that became an epidemic in Japan back in the 1950s. Methylmercury discharges into the ocean poisoned entire communities, causing disfigurement and deaths among those who were exposed to the toxin.

Some of us even know the horror stories from Medieval Europe, where things like mercury and arsenic were used in medicines—with ghastly results. Back then, mercury was used to cure syphilis, a sexually transmitted (often fatal) disease that was very common in Europe at the time. The catch? Doctors used the chloride form of mercury, which was extremely toxic and had horrible side effects. The best-case scenario was that the patient would suffer from lesions and ulcers, experience kidney failure and various neuropathies, and have their teeth fall out. The worst-case scenario (in case you still want to know), was that they'd die from mercury poisoning before the disease could get them. Talk about a lose-lose situation!

Even today, we know to be wary about mercury. Certain kinds of fish like king mackerel, swordfish, tilefish, and bigeye tuna are known to be 'high-mercury fish.' Pregnant women are told to stay away from sushi because the mercury in raw fish can cause all sorts of complications for the unborn child. So, naturally, learning that there's mercury in one's food, cosmetics, or medicine causes unspeakable alarm. But the caution, unfortunately, is often practiced in blanket terms.

In Ayurveda, most metals and minerals have some value—and this includes heavy metals like mercury, lead, and aresenic! Mercury, for example, is used in cures for viral fevers, reproductive issues, and skin problems, among others. Over the last few years, many Ayurvedic treatments have received a bad rap because of their association with heavy metals. After all, how can anything containing mercury, arsenic, or lead possibly be safe?

To understand that, let's take two factors into account:

1. Processing (shodhana or purification)

It is certainly true that taking inorganic, unprocessed mercury (or, you know, badly processed mercury, a la medieval Europe) can make you very sick. Fortunately, that's not what Ayurvedic treatments recommend you do. The processing and treatment of toxic elements is an extremely important and refined part of Ayurvedic pharmacopeia.

We already know that processing a particular element can change its physical and chemical composition completely. It can turn solids into liquids or gas. One element can be added to another to create a whole new compound that has none of the properties of the original elements. Similarly, a toxic element can be processed to make it safe for consumption. Take the example of table salt we used earlier—while chlorine is an exceedingly poisonous gas, sodium chloride is a crystalline solid that is entirely safe for consumption—obviously within limits.

Likewise, in Ayurveda, 'shodhana' is an extremely important step to be followed. Shodhana refers to any kind of purification we carry out in our day-to-day lives. For instance, to carry out shodhana of fresh milk, we boil it before we drink it. Failing to perform this step would cause us to fall ill with all the harmful bacteria that are present in the milk. It is worth noting that shodhana does not just mean cleaning, purifying, or overcoming toxic qualities of an element—it also refers to the process by which the therapeutic effects of that element are enhanced. Some methods of Shodhana include:

- Kshalana or washing
- Mardana or pounding
- Swedana or boiling
- Bhavana or levigation
- Bharjana or frying
- Nirvapa or processing in specific liquids

Different plant and mineral materials are purified in different ways, depending on their unique properties. Some purification processes call for two or more methods described here. Naturally, the shodhana of heavy metals like mercury requires one to be extremely meticulous and rigorous. It has to be done only by an expert practitioner who is trained in the process.

Ayurvedic formulations that contain mercury use a naturally occurring mercuric ore called cinnabar. Shodhana of this mercury is an elaborate process that is performed over three days. The process calls for an addition of various plant and mineral extracts in exact quantities. It requires the material to be washed and dried multiple times before it can be deemed ready for use in a therapeutic formulation. Needless to say, the end result is a form of mercury that is very different from the kind that makes up industrial effluence. Ayurvedic mercury is, in fact, the safest forms of mercury that one can use. Its therapeutic and medicinal benefits are immense. It is obviously not used in every Ayurvedic medicine out there—only very specific kinds of treatments call for the use of mercury. Purified Ayurvedic mercury, when mixed with certain plants and herbs, can act as a catalyst. It can also make the herbs more bioavailable so that they can be absorbed by your body effectively.

Likewise, there are Ayurvedic preparations that use arsenic (which is called red orpiment in its naturally occurring form) and lead (which is referred to as naga). These elements, too, have their own process of shodhana, which has to be followed before they can be rendered safe for use.

So, while Ayurvedic formulations do sometimes contain heavy metals, an educated user would know not to get alarmed simply at seeing 'mercury' or 'lead' in the label. They would know the difference between inorganic, untreated heavy metals—and their Ayurvedic counterparts that are used in these formulations. Of course, the educated user would also know better than to self-medicate or try such formulations off the counter. In the previous chapter, we talked about the role that detailed diagnosis plays in Ayurveda—medical supervision and guidance by a licensed practitioner are extremely important in any Ayurvedic treatment. To quote (or rather, translate) Acharya Charaka himself:

A potent poison also becomes the best drug on proper administration. On the contrary, even the best drug becomes a potent poison if used badly. We are seeing this sentence assume truth in a very profound way when it comes to the indiscriminate use of antibiotics.

2. Quantity

Now let's talk about the second factor that determines toxicity—quantity. Toxicity is not a black-and-white concept; nothing is unconditionally toxic or non-toxic. Dosage is extremely significant, not just in Ayurveda but in any stream of medicine under the sun.

In fact, whether we realize it or not, dosage plays an important role in our everyday life too. For instance, did you know that it is technically possible to overdose on water? Yes, the one basic thing that we all need for our body to function properly can also kill us! Drinking more water than your kidneys can process and get rid of will dilute all the electrolytes in the body—a factor that, in extreme cases, can be fatal. Don't get alarmed just yet, though. The toxic quantity of water is extremely large, and it is very difficult to drink that much water by accident. But it just goes to show that it's true what they say—too much of anything can be bad for you.

Likewise, there's a certain, minuscule quantity of chemicals and heavy metals that is also safe for your body. Since we are talking about mercury, let me give you another example of how many of us experience safe levels of exposure to it every day. For years now, dentists have used mercury in amalgam fillings. You might have some of these fillings yourself. Check your teeth—if your cavities are filled with a silvery substance, that's amalgam. It is a mixture of silver, copper, tin, and metallic mercury. Lots of people have had these fillings for years without suffering any negative health impacts. Medical research, too, has not been able to link the mercury in these fillings to any diseases. Newer fillings use resin, but that is mainly due to cosmetic reasons, as these fillings match the color of your teeth without being so conspicuous. So how are the amalgam fillings so safe despite containing mercury? The key lies in quantity. Large quantities of mercury vapor, when inhaled, can cause brain and kidney damage. But the amount of mercury used in the fillings is too small to make a difference, even if you've had them for years.

The caveat here is obvious—it is very important to determine the correct quantity of heavy metals that is safe for use, and that's a step that must be left up to licensed professionals. Dubious, unlicensed sources are not to be trusted for Ayurvedic medicines, as you can never be sure of the safety protocols they follow. As a thumb rule, the medicine you procure must be from an authentic manufacturer with a good pedigree. The facility in which it is manufactured must follow safety norms (look for the GMP or 'Good Manufacturing Practices' symbol on the product). Their Quality Assurance protocols must be fool proof—the audit trail MUST be comprehensive. The product HAS to be licensed by the Ministry of AYUSH. And importantly, do your research—and by this I don't mean just surf the internet. Obviously, Google away, but also ask around, talk to your doctor/vaidya and finally make an informed decision.

Another red flag to watch out for is if heavy metal preparations are prescribed as everyday medicines. As we discussed earlier, heavy metals are used only in certain formulations, which are then administered for very specific treatments. These medicines are usually short-term courses, with the treatment lasting from a few days to a maximum of a few months. A legitimate practitioner will never prescribe these medicines for long-term treatment except in severe cases where the benefits far outweigh the risks associated with it (think chemotherapy as an apt comparison), let alone recommend you take them as a tonic every day.

And as most fans of *Harry Potter* would know, the prescribed antidote to most poisons at Hogwarts was to shove a bezoar found in a goat's stomach down the throat of someone who ingested any poison (except, of course, that of the basilisk ☺). Now what the hell is a bezoar? Would you believe it if I said that a bezoar is a solid mass of indigestible/undigested material that accumulates in your digestive tract, sometimes causing a blockage. Bezoars usually form in the stomach, sometimes in the small intestine or, rarely, the large intestine. They can occur in children and adults. The point I am trying to make is this—don't believe everything you hear. And only half believe what you see. Make sure you understand the intricacies of what you consume. The very same principle applies to allopathy as well as Ayurveda. Get an expert to recommend the right medicine when you have a problem. YOU have no business medicating yourself or your family. Capiche?!!

Chapter 4

The Hare and the Tortoise: Myths about the Slow Action of Ayurvedic Medicines

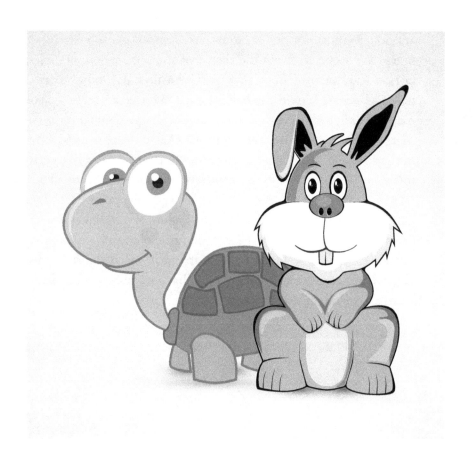

"CURING A COLD takes one week with medicine, and seven days without."

I heard this quote for the first time from a friend, back in my PhD days in the U.S. I was in the University of Utah, and if you know a thing or two about PhDs, you'll know that at times it tends to get a tad hectic. (Talk about an understatement!)

Well, this was a time when I had a massive submission due and a meeting with my advisor coming up right after. My days were mostly spent in the lab, hunched over my equipment—and when I wasn't in the lab, I was at the library, compiling my notes. I would only come home at the tail end of the day, prepare myself a quick meal and then crash out for a few hours before I had to get up and do it all over again.

The only fun thing I had on the horizon to drive me on was a hiking trip I had planned with some friends after the submissions were over. It was to be a three-day trip to Kings Peak, which is the highest point in Utah. The hike is supposed to be challenging, with some steep ridges, but the gorgeous, streaked rockface and the picture-postcard views make it all worth it. There's a beautiful lake there that we were going to camp by, before continuing our hike the next day. Needless to say, I was really looking forward to this trip.

So, when one of my friends called to say he wouldn't be able to make it, we were all pretty disappointed. What took me aback, though, was the reason he couldn't go—he had a cold. 'We still have some time before the trip. Won't you be better long before then?' I asked, surprised.

'Well, you know what they say—curing a cold takes one week with medicine and seven days without. Either way, I think I'm out for this one,' he replied.

Now, I was sad to be missing out on his company, but I was also kind of amused by this Wildean saying. I had never heard it before, but when I looked it up, I was surprised to learn that it seemed to be a common experience for many people. Most of my friends agreed to the fact that there's no real cure for the common cold—you just have to let your body fight it out.

Of course, in my experience, this 'fact' was not a fact at all. I've always known from a very young age that trifling issues like cough, cold, and fever were just that—trifling. Things that can be cured in a matter of days. I come from a pretty no-nonsense family, and coughs and colds got you out of homework and chores for a day at the most. After the medicines were administered, you'd be up and running before long. Any attempt to feign illness beyond that would only result in being disallowed from the fun stuff like playing cricket or plucking mangoes from the neighbor's trees. The homework bit, you were assured, was a safe activity since it involved sitting still for hours.

So why do I bring this up now? Well, it is to debunk a common misconception that I've often heard—that Ayurvedic treatments are very slow, and that if you want quick relief, you're better off with Western allopathic medicines. As a matter of fact, the medicines I was given as a child—the ones that cured all those colds long before the assigned one week—were all Ayurvedic formulations. This brings me to the hare-and-the-tortoise situation that defines the contrast between the two systems of medicine.

The Hare
It simply offers symptomatic relief
Now, you might be thinking of all those times when you had a fever—and how popping a quick paracetamol pill made you feel much better in half an hour or so. Can any Ayurvedic treatment possibly be faster than that? Perhaps not. So how can it be accurate to say that Ayurveda works fast?

To answer this question, let us first delve a little deeper into what fever really is. Western science defines the term 'fever' as a state when your body temperature rises above the range that is considered normal. Though it is, of course, recognized that this is a symptom of an underlying problem, the term 'fever' does not explore this in greater detail. Fever medication, thus, simply works to bring down the high temperature, thereby offering just temporary relief. Once the effects of the pill wear off, you would notice an immediate return of the temperature, the body ache, and all the other symptoms you had kept at bay. This is typically when you would take your next pill—and the cycle would continue for several days until whatever was causing the fever ran its natural course. The only other option that allopathy provides is to prevent the fever in the first place with preventive shots. Prevention, of course, is better than cure—but should you need a cure, there isn't one. Think of the common flu—you have your shots, but there's really no cure for that in allopathy. And you know you will have to get a shot again next year, because the virus continues to mutate, prompting the need for updated vaccines every time (does this sound eerily familiar to the situation we are all facing now?).

Now contrast this with the Ayurvedic term for fever—jwara. Ayurveda divides jwara into two main subtypes—'nija jwara' or jwara caused by internal factors and 'agantuja jwara' or jwara caused by external factors. These are further subdivided based on the factors causing the jwara. So, you have jwara caused by various organisms, vitiation of tissues, wounds, digestive issues, toxins, and so on. You have jwara based on seasons and other environmental factors. There are even subdivisions of jwara caused by grief, distress, or emotional turmoil. All in all, Ayurveda categorizes and defines a grand total of 64 different types of fevers!

Such precise categorization of fevers goes way back to Sushruta and Charaka's time. They had been able to isolate and identify the causes of jwara and had accordingly categorized it into the aforementioned 64 subtypes. As you can well imagine, having such precise categories makes it easy to target and treat the underlying cause that is resulting in the fever. Once the cause is identified, there are specific cures for each type of fever. So, while the symptoms may not be as quickly dealt with as in Western medicine, Ayurveda can often cure the underlying cause much faster, without having to wait for the disease to run its full course.

It is fast—but at what cost?

If you have been to any social gathering at all over the past few decades (or even just been a part of a large WhatsApp group), you would have come across that one done-to-death joke about women being bad drivers. A stereotype, obviously, but one that is so widespread, that no matter where in the world you are based, you've probably heard some version of this joke. However, did you know that men are actually way more likely to commit driving offenses and be involved in crashes? Several studies have analyzed insurance claims, crime stats, crash reports, and driving test results, and have arrived at this conclusion. (And, yes, they did take into account the fact that there are more male drivers overall. The findings hold true without exception, even after due adjustments are made.)

So why do so many people still hold on to the idea that women are worse than men behind the wheels? It may have something to do with what they consider to be 'good' driving. The studies show that men are more likely to engage in speeding, recklessness, and aggressive driving, which some may take to be a show of confidence and equate with good driving. Women, on the other hand, tend to be more cautious—which may be taken as a sign of being a 'bad' driver, of someone who is not too confident behind the wheels. This analogy, unfortunately, has a lot of parallels with many allopathic treatments.

Take liver cirrhosis. This is a condition where certain infections, diseases, and overuse of alcohol cause healthy liver cells to be damaged—and as the liver repairs itself, scar tissue forms over these damaged areas. If the damage continues and too much scar tissue forms, it becomes difficult for the liver to function normally. This has multiple, pretty serious consequences—it can cause the spleen to enlarge, one becomes unable to fight off infections effectively, and it can lead to a buildup of toxins in the brain. It increases the risk of liver cancer, and over time, it can cause multiple organs to fail. Now, as far as allopathy is concerned, liver cirrhosis cannot be reversed. It can be controlled, further damage can be checked, and associated complications can be treated. But there is no way to undo the damage to the liver and turn the scar tissues back to their healthy state. So, the only permanent cure that allopathy provides is a liver transplant.

Of course, some may consider this to be a fast cure. After all, the actual procedure takes just hours, and the patient will probably need to recover in the hospital for a couple of weeks—but after that, they're free to go, and with a brand-new liver. But, of course, it's not that simple. A liver transplant can lead to several complications like bleeding, infection, hernia, clots in the hepatic artery, and sepsis. There is a chance that the donor organ may be rejected or cause other organs to fail. And the worst part is that these worries remain, and the patient's quality of life is forever compromised. They will need to take immuno-suppressants to prevent the body from rejecting the organ, but this will hamper the body's natural ability to fight off infections. This means drastic lifestyle changes and hundreds of daily limitations and compro-mises. But as far as allopathy is concerned, this is a Hobson's choice—you either take it or leave it.

Ayurveda, however, offers a third option. Sure, the treatment may not be as quick as a couple of weeks in the hospital. But it does offer a more permanent cure—without compromising one's quality of life to that extent. The liver in Ayurveda is known as 'yakrit'—this is a literal translation of the Sanskrit phrase 'that which does.' It should come as no surprise that it is named as such because we now know that the liver is essentially the metabolic factory of the body and it performs more than 500 different functions on a daily basis. The vaidyas of yore recog-nized and understood the importance of the liver as the central organ in human health. And it is no surprise that they spent so much time and effort in being able to unravel its complexities and understanding how to remedy a damaged liver. Ayurveda has systematized the treat-ment for liver diseases to a great extent and an Ayurvedic regimen for a cirrhotic liver would consist not only of medicines for the liver but also medicines to treat the attending repercussions of a damaged liver. There are several classical formulations used to treat liver diseases. As a matter of fact, several herbs are used in judicious combinations to address a failing liver. These include but are not restricted to Punar-nava, Chitraka, Haritaki, Vibhitaki, Kalmegh, and Bhringraj. Many effective Ayurvedic liver formulations also contain metals in the form of bioavailable iron, copper, zinc, and sometimes even nanoparticles of silver. It is important to note that these are dosed appropriately after careful consideration of the patient's health status and also his genet-ics, lifestyle, and other environmental conditions. I have seen a formulation that has as many as 35 ingredients in it and the amazing part is that this in conjunction with other medicines has actually reversed liver cirrhosis in several patients. As a molecular pharmacologist with a training in biological chemistry, I find this treatment regimen to be nothing short of a high creative intelligence combined with a deep understanding of how the human body works. I am also increasingly confident that as far as liver diseases and other hard to combat life-style diseases/disorders are concerned, Ayurveda will be the new go-to solution. The cures are comprehensive and the side effects negligible to none.

The Tortoise
It is not all that slow

There are a few times in your life when you cannot afford to fall ill. The week right before your son's wedding is one of them. Yet, that's exactly what happened to Mr. Anand*. He and his wife had planned what you could call 'The Great Indian Wedding' for their son. It was to be a three-day affair, and lots of their extended family were flying in from different parts of the globe, especially to be a part of the ceremonies. Of course, their daughter-in-law-to-be had her family coming in as well—many of whom Mr. Anand would be meeting for the very first time. Welcoming a new family into your home for the first time is supposed to be an auspicious affair, and he wanted to ensure they all had a great time. But he was down with a particularly nasty strain of the flu, one that he knew would leave him in no state to be running around taking care of last-minute wedding arrangements (of which there seemed to be a thousand!).

Mr. Anand was a strong advocate of the Ayurvedic system of medi-cine and had always derived great results in the past. But this time, speed was of the essence, and more than one relative suggested he take a quick pill to suppress his symptoms and somehow go about his work. But Mr. Anand knew that was not a real solution. Plus, that way, he would risk spreading his germs to the several hundred people—guests and vendors—who were a part of the wedding. He went with his gut and reached out to our practitioners. He just had one goal—he needed to get well, and fast!

He was prescribed a combination of a classical Ayurvedic preparation called hutasini rasa, along with another formulation called sudarshana churna (which we will discuss in detail in a bit). Hutasini rasa is a preparation of processed and purified mercury in combination with Triphala, Trikatu, ginger, and purified sulfur that has extremely potent anti-viral properties, so it had good chances of working well for Mr. Anand. Besides this, our practitioners foresaw something that Mr. Anand hadn't realized yet—that his family (including his son, the groom) could already have been exposed to the virus and were at risk of falling ill too. They prescribed a combination of preventive formulations to his family. They also set up a follow-up appointment in a few days, just in case.

The treatment ended up being just right for Mr. Anand and his family. He called to cancel his follow-up appointment, saying that he had started feeling much better within two days of taking the medication. Thankfully, the rest of his family were well too, and nobody seemed to be showing any flu-like symptoms. The wedding preparations were back in full swing. Disaster averted.

This is just one of the many, many instances in which Ayurveda goes right against the popular belief of it being slow. Of course, I knew this already from personal experience, but as I researched and delved deeper into the concepts of Ayurvedic medication, I found more proof of this. Just like the tortoise in the story, medicines like hutasini rasa may not be flashy with promises of immediate relief, but it gets the job done, and done well. In the long run, it wins the race every time.

It is preventive

In December 2019, the pharmacies in Tamil Nadu noticed a strange phenomenon. They observed a sudden drop in the sale of cough and cold medicines. Autumn is usually quite a wet season in the state, and temperatures start getting a little cooler (or should I say a little less hot) toward

December. This usually means that cough, cold, and fevers run rampant through the state during this time. But in 2019, a noticeably smaller chunk of the population was falling ill. What was up?

The reason was traced to a little herb called the Andrographis paniculata, which is locally referred to as nilavembu or kalmegh. Also called the 'King of Bitters,' because of its strong taste, this plant has so many immunomodulatory and antimicrobial properties that it has been used for a wide array of treatments for hundreds of years. And I really do mean a wide array. From the common cold and sinusitis to conditions like arthritis, eczema, and even high blood pressure—nilavembu has curative properties to treat all these and more. More recently, a concoction of the nilavembu along with eight other herbs had been found to not only prevent but also cure chikungunya and treat dengue. Both diseases are pretty widespread in tropical places like Tamil Nadu, especially in the monsoon—and so far, neither has an allopathic cure.

Knowing its effectiveness against these diseases, the Tamil Nadu government had started distributing a concoction of nilavembu to people across the state, free of cost. As it turned out, its preventive properties extended to even the common cough, cold, and fevers, and it ended up keeping a huge percentage of the population healthy through the monsoon. So much so, that it was actually bringing down the sales of some of the common medicines!

However, there's one statement that I would like to add here, and it's one that I have mentioned before—any Ayurvedic treatment is best taken after consultation with a licensed practitioner. The science of preparing Ayurvedic formulations is a precise one, and the same treatment may work differently on different people. An Ayurvedic practitioner will help you ensure that whatever formulation you are taking is right and safe for you.

It can tackle a variety of diseases at once
If you are familiar with Hindu mythology, you would know about Lord Vishnu's Sudarshana Chakra. If not, look up any image of Lord Vishnu or his incarnation as Lord Krishna, and you will see him depicted with a

wheel or disk with serrated edges balanced on his forefinger. This disk is called the Sudarshana Chakra and it is considered to be the most formidable weapon wielded by any God in Hindu mythology.

Unlike any regular weapon that needs to be thrown or brandished, the Sudarshana Chakra is wielded with the power of Lord Vishnu's will alone. When Lord Vishnu wills it to be sent against some evil force, the disk leaves his finger, spinning at an astounding speed and covering massive distances in the blink of an eye—and it doesn't stop until it finds its target and decimates it. As one of the deadliest weapons in the entire cosmos, it is said to have the power to destroy all evil that comes before it—it is the ultimate force of order and preservation.

So, when you hear of a medicine that is named after the Sudarshana Chakra, you can rightly expect it to be something extraordinary. And the sudarshana churna doesn't disappoint.

This classical formulation is prepared using a combination of an astounding 43–54 ingredients, based on which treatise one is referring to. For instance, the *Bhaisajya Ratnavali* (one of the classical textbooks that all Ayurvedic vaidyas have in their library) lists out 43 ingredients for the preparation of sudarshana churna, while the *Yoga Ratnakara* (a compendium that embeds in its pages all Ayurvedic knowledge up to the 17th century) recommends 54. The difference may have been due to the fact that certain plants were only available in specific regions of India. The *Sahasrayogam*, which is a text from Kerala dating back to the mid-20th century, collates different methods of preparation from different parts of the country—and it recommends 49 ingredients. However, as per the AYUSH Ministry of India, all three texts are valid references for the legitimate manufacturing of medicines.

Irrespective of which treatise one follows, the process for preparing sudarshana churna is very detailed and precise. The herbs need to be cleaned, dried in the shade, sorted, ground to a precise degree, and mixed into one homogenous mass. The final result is a yellowish-brown, bitter powder that has been proven to have anti-inflammatory, antipyretic, analgesic, antiviral, antibacterial, antifungal, antioxidant, hepatoprotective, antidiabetic, anti-asthmatic, antitussive, immunomodulatory, and antidiarrheal properties. An astounding portfolio of curative capabilities!

This medicine wards off most disease-causing organisms and is known to target and treat any and every disease that has fever as one of its symptoms, which, in itself, is quite an achievement when you consider the 64 different types of jwara (fever) we discussed earlier. To appreciate the significance of this, think about whether a paracetamol tablet can do this. Imagine you contract a throat infection and run a high fever as an associated symptom. A paracetamol tablet will only bring down your fever for a few hours, but the infection will remain. To cure this, you will need to go to a doctor, who will probably prescribe a strong course of antibiotics. Until you finish that course and shake off the infection once and for all, the fever will keep coming back. Not so with the sudarshana churna. Just like Lord Vishnu's daunting weapon that finds its evil target and doesn't rest until it has been destroyed, this classical Ayurvedic formulation seeks out the root of the fever and treats it, thereby tackling the cause and the symptom all in one go.

This is one medicine that has proved its worth to a great extent in the context of the COVID-19 pandemic. Ours is an organization that operates under the essential services industry—given that we prepare medicines (and in recent times, hand sanitizers), we could not afford to stay home and shelter in place. But it was also important to ensure that everyone in the organization remained well protected as they came to work every day. We relied on the sudarshana churna formulation to ward off diseases and build up our immunity—with the result that not one person in the organization showed any symptoms.

It offers cures for things you don't expect to have a cure for

A few years back, Divya* came to us for a consultation with our Ayurvedic specialists. Divya was just 13 or 14 years old at the time, and she suffered from a peculiar condition (one that she had had ever since she was a little girl). Every morning, she would wake up with a runny nose. And I'm not talking about your everyday sniffles either—she would actually go through four or five handkerchiefs before she left for school. Most of us would call in sick if we woke up feeling that bad, but since it was an everyday affair for Divya, she had no choice but to power through. Needless to say, it wasn't a very pleasant experience for her, but no doctor had been able to identify the issue or offer a cure, so she struggled through this all throughout her childhood. As she grew older, her workload at school grew more challenging. And it didn't end with the school day either—she had her music practice after school, and from there, she'd have to head to her coaching classes a few days a week, where she was getting some extra help with certain subjects. Unfortunately, all this was getting a little too much for her body to cope with given that her mornings made her feel tired and worn out before the day even began. That's when her parents brought her to us for help.

After a detailed observation, we concluded that it was a form of allergy that's triggered in the mornings. This diagnosis helped us chart out a course of treatments for her. We prescribed a combination of medicines from our arsenal, and within a few days, she started noticing an improvement. A month or so down the line, she was perfectly fine. By this, I mean that she was able to stop taking the medicines altogether, without reverting to her previous state.

This recovery wasn't miraculous. Nor was it some kind of fluke. In allopathy, allergies are treated as a fact of life. There is no real, permanent cure for them—you are just expected to accept the fact and move on, trying to avoid whatever you are allergic to for the rest of your life. The best you can do is pop an antihistamine pill that will suppress your reaction to the trigger. Lots of people go through their entire lives being allergic to dust, hay, pollution, or pollen. The last one is particularly brutal—imagine suffering from allergies for an entire season at a time.

Ayurveda, however, has options to not just treat or suppress the symptoms, but offer a permanent cure. Allergies are nothing but disorders of the immune system. Certain irritants cause the immune system to trigger hypersensitive reactions that manifest in different ways—sneezing, breathing difficulties, nasal secretions, or tears. An Ayurvedic course of medicines will be tailored specifically to your triggers, your reactions, and your particular body composition. And, of course, by now, you should have guessed it—food takes a prime position in the whole treatment regimen. For example, dairy is a trigger that most people are not aware of, especially if you consume non-A2 milk-based dairy. The kind of foods one consumes also plays a very important role in addressing your allergies. Light and warm food is preferred over heavy and cold foods like meats and others. You will in all likelihood be recommended for an Ayurvedic cleanse known as panchakarma. Post this, medicines will be prescribed. Typically, you start seeing a difference in a few weeks or so—which may be slower than the immediate results that an antihistamine will give you, but once again, it is a cure that is very permanent. Once your course is over, your body will no longer react to pollen (or dust, hay, fibers, etc.) the same way.

*Names changed to protect identity

CHAPTER 5

The Gourmand's Curse: Myths Associated with Dietary Practices in Ayurveda

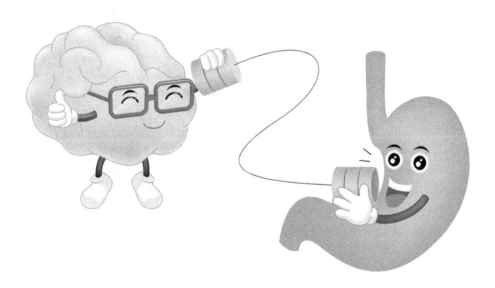

IT WAS ONE of my least favorite days of the month. It was Dwadashi. Why was that so bad? Well, it meant that I could tell you with my eyes closed what would be on the menu that day. Boiled mung lentils tempered with ginger. A vegetable preparation made with amaranth leaves. Rasam, which is a light, almost watery lentil soup seasoned with different spices. Even the sweet dish would be a kind of pudding prepared with boiled mung beans. The ten-year-old me hated it. And the most annoying bit? Dwadashi comes around every fortnight, which means that these items would be on the table once every two weeks, without fail.

The young gourmand in me protested (as loudly as he dared) at this recurring gastronomical ordeal. Of course, I did not yet understand the implication of Dwadashi, let alone get why it merited this bland fare. And if you are not familiar with the traditional Hindu lunar calendar either, let me explain.

Dwadashi literally means 'the twelfth day.' It follows Ekadashi, the eleventh day, which traditionally was a day of fasting. Yes, the ancient vedic system that our ancestors followed (from which Ayurveda emerged) prescribed a day of fasting on the eleventh day of every fortnight. This was done to eliminate toxins and undigested food materials accumulated in the body. A cleanse if you will.

Of course, being too young, I was not expected to fast—but all the adults in the household did follow this schedule rigorously. And just like there's a right way to fast, Ayurveda also sets out the right way to break a fast. You cannot just jump in and indulge in a rich fry-up or lots of caffeine. Not eating anything for 24 hours sparks off certain chemical reactions in your digestive system and causes a lot of gasses to build up. A heavy, greasy, or overly spicy meal will only aggravate this and make you feel terrible the rest of the day. So, you ease in with a lighter fare, making sure to include things like mung, ginger and amaranth greens, which are known to negate and tackle the gasses in your body. Having observed the Ekadashi fast, my family needed this meal every fortnight. Of course, I did not know this then. Indeed, my family did not follow this as a part of some specific Ayurvedic lifestyle—they were just following a centuries-old tradition, doing as their parents had done. It was only when I grew up and studied biological chemistry and understood the processes that happen inside the body that I appreciated the logical merit of this system. Once I understood the need for it, this traditional fortnightly meal was much easier to swallow (both literally and metaphorically!).

Food, Fuel, and Fads

Here, in this chapter, I want to discuss Ayurveda and its strong ties with dietary practices. The overarching sentiment that I have heard way too many times when it comes to Ayurveda is that the system poses too many dietary restrictions that are too rigorous and limiting. At first glance, some of these may seem to be based entirely on traditional beliefs and religious practices. However, as one delves deeper into Ayurvedic recommendations, it becomes more obvious that they have their roots solidly planted in medical science. That was certainly the case with me and the Dwadashi menu!

And if you are wondering about the legitimacy of a fortnightly fast in the first place, let me introduce you to Yoshinori Ohsumi. He is a Japanese cell biologist who was awarded the Nobel Prize in 2016 for his work on autophagy. Autophagy is a process of cell renewal that occurs during phases of starvation. During this process, cells break down proteins, cell components, and other damaged structures for energy—and bacteria and viruses are also destroyed in this process. So, what triggers this autophagy? Would you believe it—fasting for 12–24 hours?

It is no surprise that fasting is a part of many ancient cultures, including the system of Ayurveda. There are many such examples of Ayurvedic practices turning out to have deep-rooted scientific explanations, which were only proved by formal studies in recent years. The logical basis of these practices becomes clearer the more one explores the system.

But what about the rigor and limitations of Ayurvedic diets? Let's break this statement into two parts and discuss each in turn.

The Rigor

We live in an age of diets and food restrictions—that's just a truth universally acknowledged. Just think of the last dinner party you hosted for a mixed group of friends. Apart from the usual vegetarian and non-vegetarian options, you may have had to keep in mind that some of your guests were following specific diet plans—vegan, paleo, or keto. Others may have had certain food allergies to negotiate, so you may have needed to ensure that there were enough gluten-free, dairy-free, and nut-free options. And that's the truth of our lifestyles—even though these specifications and diet restrictions are not necessarily easy, lots of people are willing to follow them (often voluntarily) over the long term because they understand their benefits. And the longer they follow the practices, the more a part of their lifestyles they become, getting easier over time. The mindset you need to embrace an Ayurvedic diet is no different. It might even be a tad easier because here you can rest assured that you are not following a fad diet—you are taking on something that has been tried and tested for thousands of years.

In fact, a lot of the newer diet plans you hear about actually promote theories that have been presented and followed by Ayurvedic vaidyas centuries ago. Take the intermittent fasting pattern, which breaks your day into cyclic phases of eating and fasting. One of the most popular recommendations under this plan is the 16:8 method—that's when you fast for 16 hours, and then have all your meals in the following eight-hour window. And it's not that difficult either if you think about it—it just involves skipping your breakfast. If you have your first meal at 11:00 a.m. and finish the last one by 7:00 p.m., that's intermittent fasting. This pattern essentially just gives your body more time to absorb the food you have consumed, and there's enough research out there to show that when done right, it can improve metabolism and help your body become leaner and more muscular.

Now, let's consider the fact that ancient Ayurvedic diets did not have a concept of breakfast as a big meal. Ayurveda only prescribed two meals a day—lunch and supper, taken within a few hours of each other. Sounds familiar?

Of course, there's a wrong way to carry out intermittent fasting too, which can quickly take it from a useful practice to just another fad. If you're only indulging in junk food in the 'eating hours,' or you're blindly following it without taking your lifestyle or any underlying health issues into account, then it can do more harm than good. But if you actually do it right, and with proper guidance, then it can work wonders. The key lies in how you follow it. For instance, the first couple of days you might be tempted to gorge yourself at 11:00 a.m. when you break the fast. Then around 4:00 p.m., you binge again. By 7:00 p.m., you might find that you're not all that hungry—so you end up NOT being able to optimize your window of eating hours. Soon enough, you start feeling hungry later at night, and this new diet seems way too 'trendy' and difficult.

Pretty soon, you'd realize that a better way to go about it would be to eat a normal meal at 11:00 a.m., perhaps have some lighter snacks at 4:00 p.m., and then finish the day with another decent meal at 7:00 p.m. And that's just what Ayurveda would tell you to do in the first place. Not just that, it will also nudge you toward the kinds of food that will be healthier for you, satiate your hunger, and keep you full longer. So, overall, an Ayurvedic diet might actually be easier to follow!

The belief that these restrictions are specific to Ayurveda

Of course, lifestyle and personal values are not the only reason you might follow a certain diet. Sometimes, it might actually be medically mandated by your doctor. And there we arrive at another important point when it comes to food. Dietary restrictions are not just a part of Ayurvedic medicine—Western and allopathic medical systems have them too. Indeed, there isn't a single medical system that will just give you free rein to binge on whatever you please.

Let's talk allopathy. You might already know that many of the most common diseases today arise from poor dietary practices. Of course, there are genetic components to diseases too, but diet- and lifestyle-led diseases are much more frequent in occurrence. Let's take some of the most common ailments of today and look at how they affect one's diet.

- **Diabetes**: While Type 1 diabetes is genetic, Type 2 diabetes is lifestyle-driven and very preventable. An allopathic doctor would know that simply prescribing medicines would not suffice—they will recommend several kinds of food restrictions for diabetic patients too. For example, someone suffering from diabetes might be asked to avoid complex carbohydrates like white rice, processed grains, and refined flour. Obesity and accumulation of belly fat have major correlations with diabetes, so the patient might be asked to watch their calorie intake throughout the day. They might need to eliminate starchy foods like potatoes, full-fat dairy products, red meats, cheeses, and butter. Of course, sugary foods like cakes, cookies, ice-creams, and fizzy drinks will likely be off the table too—quite literally. Instead, the patient might be asked to incorporate lots of vegetables, leafy greens, lean proteins, and healthy grains like brown rice, barley, and millets.

- **Heart disease:** Saturated trans fats and high levels of "bad" cholesterol have been linked to heart disease, so these are probably the first things an allopathic doctor will ask a patient to cut out. This would automatically eliminate all sorts of fried and fast foods. In addition, it will also involve minimizing the consumption of red meats like beef and pork, as well as processed meats. Packaged, preserved, and canned foods often contain high levels of sodium and sugar, so they might be restricted as well. Just like with diabetic patients, heart patients too will be asked to have more whole foods, veggies, and greens. A thumb rule that cardiologists usually follow is to recommend that vegetables comprise at least 50 percent of one's meal.
- **Obesity:** Obesity in itself can lead to a whole host of other health issues and complications. So, bringing the patient's weight back to a medically approved level will be the top priority for the doctor. A ketogenic diet is often recommended these days, as this has been shown to be effective in weight loss. This is a low-carb diet that's high in fat followed by proteins. This might seem counter-intuitive at first glance, but it basically prompts your body to burn fat for fuel instead of the usual carbs. This high metabolic state is called ketogenesis. To achieve this, one needs to avoid breads, pastas, chocolates, and sugary sodas (surprise, surprise). But also, most fruits, beans, lentils, and some veggies will have to be eliminated—which might come as a shock, since these are usually considered to be healthy.

The point is that dietary restrictions and medicine always go hand in hand, and you can seldom have just the latter without the former. So why are dietary restrictions posed by Ayurveda considered to be difficult and limiting while there is an air of inevitability and acceptance when it comes to restrictions suggested by allopathy? Well, maybe because people only seek (allopathic) medical help once something has gone wrong and it has become obvious to the patient that a dietary and lifestyle overhaul might be required. Ayurveda is more holistic and deals more with the prevention of diseases in the first place. But before something is actually wrong, it might be difficult to recognize the need for a healthy diet. The mindset is the only thing that is different—the actual diet, I promise you, is no more difficult than any restriction an allopathic doctor might propose.

The Ayurvedic Approach

Now that we have established that (a) Ayurvedic dietary restrictions are no more rigorous than any other diet you might follow, and (b) other medical systems have their own dietary restrictions too, let's come to the specifics of nutrition in Ayurveda. Why should you follow this particular system instead of just taking your pick from any other diet plan you find online? Or indeed, why not wait for your doctor to suggest one? Well, here are just a few reasons to get you started.

1. **It takes a personalized approach**

    One of the reasons why choosing and following a particular diet is so difficult is because of the sheer volume of information out there. Just do a quick search on diets to help you lose weight (or put on muscle mass or have more energy—really, just insert any health goal here). You'll immediately be inundated with thousands of articles, all giving you a variety of tips and tricks, some of which will be quite contradictory. Some might recommend a low-carb diet to lose weight, another one will claim you need to amp up your fat intake, and yet another will recommend various cleanses. There will be celebrities endorsing miraculous powders and smoothies. Some fitness instructors will claim that it's impossible to bulk up unless you have steaks for every meal; others will insist that you haven't lived until you've embraced veganism. And every one of them will have data, stats, and anecdotes to prove that they are right.

But they can't all be right, can they? How can vast amounts of contradictory data all be true? Surely someone's fudging the truth. While I won't pretend that everything you read on the internet is true (it definitely is not, and that Nigerian prince is not looking for someone to leave all his wealth to either!), there is a way that contradictory reports can be legitimate. The answer lies in uniqueness— what works for you may not work for another person, and vice versa.

An important concept that one must remember is that it's not just Ayurvedic medicine that is personalized—the Ayurvedic diet is too. Every one of us has very different body compositions and constitutions, so we cannot expect our bodies to thrive on cookie-cutter diets. Ayurvedic diets take into account your 'prakriti,' which basically means the physical and physiological aspects that make you unique. It also keeps in mind your lifestyle, genetic markers, and even psychological factors. Do note that two people with very similar genetic makeup and environmental circumstances can also have vastly different prakritis and therefore, need different diets. For example, a diet without rice makes me feel more energetic while it just doesn't work for my brother—it makes him feel tired and fatigued, even if he's had a wholesome meal otherwise. Moreover, an Ayurvedic diet is also personalized based on changing seasons, times of the day, and your geographical location. If you are seeking treatment for some disease, then your practitioner will carry out a careful diagnosis, following the processes we have discussed previously. They will then recommend the ideal diet for you, which will keep your specifications in mind and complement the treatment you are prescribed.

Many of these parameters are conspicuously absent from allopathic and trending diets. For instance, you might notice that when a diet becomes popular, people all around the world hasten to embrace it, irrespective of whether they live in a balmy city like Chennai or a cold place like Ottawa. This explains why fad diets often don't work. This also explains why one celebrity may claim to feel their best with a high-protein diet while another swears carbs are the best for sustained health. It does not say anything about the diets per se—it simply means that both celebrities were lucky enough to have found what works best for them.

2. It makes no sweeping statements

When I look at the diet plans out there today, I am shocked by the sweeping declarations that some of them make. Ingredients, components, and even entire food groups are decisively termed as 'good' or 'bad' with nary a disclaimer or a caveat in sight. But what about the studies, the proponents would protest. And it's true—there are volumes of research papers and legitimate studies to show that this, that, and the other claim is true. People tend to reject empirical evidence based on the fact that there is no formal proof—but give them a research paper, and suddenly they are willing to take a lot more information at face value.

What many people do not realize, however, is that the very nature of research is evolutionary. New information comes to light every year, that may completely disprove what was believed before. A few chapters back, we discussed the egg yolk and the demonization of cholesterol. Now we know that not every kind of cholesterol is bad. A few decades before this, there was widespread panic about monosodium glutamate (MSG), with experts linking it to everything from autism and Alzheimer's disease to depression, obesity, and cancer. None of these studies, however, were conclusive. Today, we see a similar response to gluten, with thousands of people who do not suffer from Celiac disease shunning gluten en masse (by the way, if you have celiac disease, you certainly must avoid gluten. The reason is that gluten triggers a series of pathways with molecules having names that sound like alien species from *Star Trek* (gliadin and zonulin if you actually wanted to know) that eventually lead to a leaky gut, which leads to inflammation, which triggers the various symptoms associated with celiac disease. And of course, there are longer running discourses that we are all familiar with. Is wine good or bad? What about coffee? Is it ok to give sugar to children?

The truth is that it is extremely difficult to carry out nutritional research in a way that completely eliminates emotions, biases, and subjectivity. There is the placebo effect to take into account. There's also the expectation bias—in the studies on MSG, many test subjects responded negatively to it because they genuinely believed they were intolerant and exaggerated its effects in their mind. Most of these studies also rely on self-reporting, where test subjects have to remember what they ate and how they reacted to those foods. Needless to say, it's not always accurate.

Ayurveda acknowledges and understands that these discourses are more nuanced. Its personalized approach alone means that the practice cannot slot anything as 'good' or 'bad' in absolute terms— because as discussed earlier, what's bad for one person may be suitable for another. Alternatively, what's bad for you in one season may be good for you in another season and under other circumstances. Similarly, statements like 'the human digestive system is not meant to process dairy' (or grains or meat) may sound scientific, but are not always true. People have, after all, been consuming these things for centuries, and any negative fallouts are likely to apply to a select few rather than the entire human race! A legitimate Ayurvedic practitioner will never make these kinds of sweeping declarations you may come across online.

Here's another common example. Ayurveda typically recommends a diet rich in plant sources. But if you are into sports or fitness, you might have been told time and again that a vegetarian diet is unhealthy for you as it can never give you the kind of proteins you need for muscle repair. This is, again, untrue. You can definitely get all the required proteins from plant sources—there are enough examples of elite athletes and sportspersons who excel on plant-based diets.

However, a wide variety of veggies will be prescribed to ensure you get all the amino acids you need. A single type of vegetable is unlikely to suffice, no matter how much of a superfood it is claimed to be.

3. **It is well balanced**

Speaking of varied diets, it is interesting to note that Ayurveda makes space for all kinds of foods. Of course, it does leverage the goodness of whole foods, grains, fruits, and vegetables as much as possible. But here again, the system challenges some of the common perceptions we have today.

Firstly, we are programmed to think of raw foods as something good. After all, a salad is the healthiest thing you can have, right? Well, not quite. Common nutritional disquisition states that cooking causes vegetables to lose a lot of the essential nutrients that are naturally contained within. However, Ayurveda promotes the consumption of only cooked foods. The concept of bioavailability comes into play here. While raw vegetables may indeed have more nutrients, they are not too easy to digest—so our bodies may have trouble breaking them down to optimize all these nutrients. Cooked food, however, is easily broken down by our enzymes, so it ensures better absorption of nutrients. Cooking also allows us to make optimum use of spices. An Ayurvedic diet will typically incorporate all the six flavors or 'rasas' (sweet, sour, bitter, salty, astringent, and pungent) into each meal, though the dominant flavors will change depending on your prakriti.

Secondly, on the flip side of the coin, we are also programmed to think of certain foods as inherently bad. Think meats, fats, and alcohol. The Ayurvedic nutritional approach, however, includes all of these. Let's take a look at the *Charaka Samhita*. During autumn or 'hemanta,' Charaka suggests, 'One should use the unctuous, sour and salted juice of the meat of dominantly fatty and aquatic and marshy animals, and also the meat of burrow-dwelling animals. After this, the person should drink wine, vinegar, and honey. One does not lose lifespan if he takes regularly milk products, cane sugar, fats, oil, new rice, and hot water during hemanta.' Likewise, the meat of hare, antelope, quail, and partridge are also recommended in certain seasons and as a restorative cure for certain ailments. Again, this is not for everyone. It is recommended that this be the diet for someone who is involved in rigorous activity, lives in a cold place, has a particular type of physiology, his/her disease state and so forth. While Ayurveda does not support animal cruelty, it does not promote veganism either. Meat consumption occupies a very small part of the Ayurvedic diet, but ghee, honey, and dairy products have important roles to play in this nutritional system.

Of course, it is important to note that while an Ayurvedic diet includes all kinds of food, it does not give one blanket permission to eat anything, anytime. Be it plants, meats, legumes, or alcohol, the system puts forward specific guide-lines for consumption. It outlines the ideal season and time of day to consume each item. Quantity is obviously important too, so the diet will include specific portion sizes. Another unique aspect of this diet is its acknowledgment of food incompat-ibilities. Your practitioner may ask you not to combine certain foods or have them together in large quantities. For example, combining too many sour fruits and dairy products is generally discouraged due to their incompatible natures. In general, fruits and milk are not to be combined as per Ayurveda (there goes your fruit-based milkshake, eh!?)

4. **It is holistic**

Today, we are all too used to multi-tasking, and unfortunately, this extends to our dietary practices as well. Ever had lunch at your desk and been so focused on your work that you barely noticed what you ate? Ever been so engrossed in a Netflix show that you polished off an entire bag of chips without even realizing it?

What you eat and how much you eat is important in Ayurveda of course—but so is how you eat. After all, food is not just something you have for its nutritional properties alone. It is also meant to be enjoyed and savored; it is meant to satiate you mentally.

An Ayurvedic diet brings one back to mindful eating practices. It recommends that you maintain regular eating habits, having your meals at the same hours each day, without skipping meals or snacking at odd times. It also suggests that you sit down for your meals on a raised surface, according to Sushruta. This is the exact opposite of what the world, at large, practices today. Nowadays, the food is at a higher level than your seat. In fact, my family continues to eat the way it is recommended. We sit on a raised plank while the plate containing the food is on the clean floor), rather than eating it on the go. In fact, it discourages any kind of distraction while eating, thus enabling you to savor each bite and truly enjoy the smell, taste, and texture of food. Moreover, it allows you to pay closer attention to your body's signals that indicate when you are full. This is an important cue that distracted eaters often miss, which results in overeating. Sushruta also recommends a short walk after meals.

5. **It does not claim to be the cure-all for all ills**
'Let food be thy medicine and medicine be thy food.'

This is a quote that is often attributed to Hippocrates, who is known as the father of (western) medicine. If at all you are interested in health and fitness (or have friends on social media who are), you have almost certainly come across this quote. While the sentiment expressed here certainly rings true with Ayurveda too, such statements are often misinterpreted in some pretty extreme ways.

Some people go into it blindly, believing that a sudden change in food habits will magically cure any and every disease they are suffering from. There are heartbreaking accounts of people who refused to seek treatment for diseases like cancer, choosing instead to take a dietary approach to tackle their ills. As you may have guessed, these stories do not have a happy ending. Others treat the sentiment with strong cynicism. They think this is a top way in which 'alternate medicine' exploits gullible believers. And indeed, I am sure that there are many unscrupulous practitioners, miracle workers, and quacks who do promise impossible results.

While I don't claim to know about every scam that's out there, what I can do is make sure you know what the Ayurvedic nutritional system can and cannot do. Hopefully, this will help people distinguish legitimate Ayurvedic nutritional knowledge from random exploitative scams.

Ayurveda does believe that most of the diseases we suffer from today are caused by poor dietary practices. Obviously, there are diseases that are nor related to diet like COVID-19 (oh wait . . . didn't the whole thing start because some bat-eating jackass in Wuhan, China, decided to succumb to his gastro-nomical cravings!?) and other infectious diseases like typhoid, malaria, cholera, dengue, etc. However, once a disease has been contracted, diet alone cannot and should not be used in lieu of proper medical attention. If that was the case, then there would be no need for Ayurvedic treatments and therapies either— one could just eat oneself better. But as it stands, treatments, medicines, and in some cases, surgery, all have their place in this medical system.

However, when it comes to prevention, your diet can go a long, long way. As we saw earlier, ailments like heart disease, diabetes, and obesity have their roots in poor dietary and lifestyle choices—and these, in turn, lead to various other complications. A well moderated, balanced diet that is tailored to your constitution can help you prevent these ailments. When it comes to more mundane illnesses like colds, flus, and fevers, your diet can help build up your immunity and prevent you from falling ill every time you are exposed to any bacteria or virus.

The other advantage an Ayurvedic diet gives you is in recuperation. It can help you recover from various illnesses more effectively, and in many cases, it can even reverse the harmful impacts of the disease. For example, in the case of COVID-19, many patients complain of general weakness after being tested negative. Along with the proper nourishment in terms of food, Ayurvedic rasayanas and formulations that contain zinc nanoparticles, borax nanoparticles, gokshuradi churna (a magnificent mix of Tribulus terrestris and eight other ingredients), calcium nanoparticles, ashwagandha, and shatavari, patients have been able to shrug off this rather irritating and debilitating general weakness in an extraordinarily effective manner. When used in conjunction with the right treatment, Ayurveda can help you bounce back faster and prevent relapses.

Ayurveda and Immunity

Immunity—that's one aspect of our health that many of us had all but forgotten until the coronavirus pandemic reminded us with a sudden, rude jolt. Most systems of medicine are reactive. They cure diseases that one has already contracted or provide vaccines for diseases that we are already familiar with. But what happens when a sudden mutation of a virus causes a new disease that we have neither a vaccine nor a cure for? Global lockdowns, worldwide panic, and countless lives lost.

The COVID-19 pandemic has reminded us that perhaps it is not such a great idea to lead unwholesome lifestyles and then depend completely on medicines when something goes wrong. Perhaps it is smart to prep our own systems in such a way that our bodies are able to ward off diseases on their own, without putting all the pressure on our medical systems. Perhaps it is time to make immunity a priority.

Our immune system is our biological defense to diseases and infections. We are constantly exposed to different microbes and pathogens as

we go about our day-to-day lives. A healthy immune system is able to identify and attack these pathogens as they enter your body, destroying them
before they make you ill. In most cases, it will also develop a resistance to
those pathogens, thereby protecting you from that particular disease in
the future too.

However, the immune system does not function like this unconditionally. It needs to be maintained and augmented in order for it to work at
optimum levels. We discussed earlier in the chapter that the Ayurvedic
system of medicine traces most diseases back to improper digestion and
the diets we follow. While at first glance, this may seem like an over-
simplification of complex issues, this basically refers to the fact that the
immune system is intrinsically linked to the food we eat. Unwholesome
diets, irregular timings, and other improper habits cause a build-up of
undigested food materials (referred to as 'ama') in the body, which makes
the immune system sluggish and inadequate.

But the good news is, this also means that the reverse is true—our
food habits and dietary practices can also help boost the immune system
and keep it functioning optimally, which in turn prevents and wards off
diseases. This is where the Ayurvedic concept of 'ojas' comes in. Just like
improperly digested food produces ama, ojas is what you get when the
food you consume is metabolized properly by your body. You know the
sparkling eyes, luscious locks, and healthy glow that some people have,
that no amount of makeup can replicate? That's a sign of high levels of ojas
being produced in the body. Sufficient levels of ojas boost the immune
system, create resistance and resilience against diseases, and keep the different systems well balanced.

An Ayurvedic diet can help you understand the kinds of food
that will keep your body healthy and robust. It will include a good
balance of carbohydrates, proteins and vitamins, minerals and good
fats, all seasoned with a hearty mix of spices. I have already talked
about how Ayurvedic diets incorporate all the six flavors (sweet,
sour, bitter, salty, astringent, and pungent) in each meal. This is not
done for variety alone. Spices in Ayurveda don't just add flavor—

their role goes much beyond that. Different flavors are known to trigger the production of different digestive enzymes in your body, which help you digest your food better, thereby promoting the creation of ojas. Spices are also recognized to boost immunity and have valuable therapeutic properties. If you want to know exactly how much spices can do, just refer to the box in the next few pages. You'll be surprised and amazed at how many everyday issues they can help you solve!

Little Known Superpowers of Everyday Spices

Ginger: Ginger has so many curative properties, that it is referred to as a 'maha aushudha' in Ayurveda—which basically means super drug! You probably already know that ginger helps you get rid of coughs, colds, and gas. But did you know that it can also help you get rid of that throbbing earache? All you need to do is crush some ginger to extract the juice, and then just pour a few drops in your ears. Crushed ginger paste, when applied to your forehead, can also get rid of headaches. And if you're looking to cut down on coffee, you can mix equal parts of ginger, honey, and lemon juice. Just one spoonful of this mix helps you get rid of drowsiness.

Curry leaves: This is great for digestion, has fantastic anti-diabetic properties, and when consumed regularly in food, it is good for the liver too. And if you suffer from motion sickness but are tired of the medicines that knock you out cold for hours, curry leaves can come to the rescue. Simply dry the leaves, crush them into a fine powder, and mix four portions of it with one portion of cardamom for an effective motion sickness remedy. Curry leaf powder mixed with honey is a great cure for mouth ulcers too.

Coriander: Coriander powder, when used in food, prevents bloating and gas. Don't forget to temper your food with coriander seeds

---

either—regular consumption can promote hair growth and delay balding patterns.

Cumin: This is another great spice to use in food, as it is a rich source of iron, zinc, and vitamin C, and can help boost your immune system. And if you are trying to quit smoking or alcohol consumption, try chewing on some ground cumin powder whenever you get the cravings. Cumin has been proven to be really effective in kicking addictions and drug dependencies.

Cloves: Everyone knows about the immunity-boosting properties of cloves and their uses in soothing nausea and toothaches. But did you know they can help you get rid of those annoying hiccups too? Pop a clove into your mouth, and the hiccups will be gone in no time. Chewing one clove a day can also help improve eyesight.

Black pepper: This has its uses in heart complaints and acts as a fantastic stomach cleanser. But you may not have known how helpful it is in clearing chest congestions too. Just chew a mixture of black pepper powder, honey, and betel leaves before bed. The next morning, the phlegm in your chest will be expelled in the form of a productive cough.

Fennel: If you regularly suffer from terrible pre-menstrual syndrome (PMS) symptoms and debilitating cramps during your periods, fennel can be extremely helpful for you. Having fennel regularly has been shown to reduce these cramps over time. Of course, fennel is good for treating worm infestation and constipation too.

Cardamom: If you suffer from bad breath, try chewing some cardamom instead of gum. Cardamom triggers your salivary glands, thereby getting rid of the dryness in your mouth and the subsequent odor. A fine powder of cardamom can also be given to children who suffer from painful urination in the summer.

Cinnamon: Not just great for flavoring your coffee and baked goods, cinnamon helps you get rid of headaches too. Instead of reaching for an aspirin the next time, try chewing a small bark of cinnamon, letting the extract flow into your stomach. That headache will be gone before long.

Turmeric: Of course, turmeric is currently enjoying its moment in the spotlight, so most people have already heard of its many curative properties. But here are a couple you may not have heard of yet. Applying turmeric to your skin will not just help you prevent breakouts, it can slow hair growth too. Also, if you suffer from sinus, try burning a turmeric rhizome and inhaling the fumes. It can help soothe those brutal headaches right away.

I will reiterate here that this kind of diet is not a fad or a passing trend, although some aspects of it are trending right now. While modern experts are realizing and advocating the benefits of fats and spices in your diet now, these practices have been followed for thousands of years in India. Indian traditional cooking is actually one of the best in the world, in terms of the sheer range of ingredients and spices it incorporates into everyday meals.

Apart from the varied ingredients used in foods, Ayurveda also recommends drinking different kinds of teas, infusions, and of course, plenty of water throughout the day. Moreover, it may prescribe certain herbal powders and extracts that will help you process your food well. Paired with mindful eating practices, regular fasting, and detox schedules (like the Ekadashi fast my family follows), the diet takes care of every aspect of your digestion. Done right, it can be all you need to get your immune system back at the top of its game, so that the next time you come in contact with some kind of germ (be it something simple like the common cold or something more complex), your body will be able to shake it right off without you even realizing it.

If it's true that you are what you eat, an Ayurvedic diet ensures that you are healthy, tough, and incredibly vigorous. The importance of diet and its effect on gut bacteria and the subsequent cascading results that the gut microbiome (microbiome is a term for the entire set of microorganisms found in the body) has on human health has led to the blossoming of a new branch of science called 'Microbiomics.' Indeed, there is an ever-growing body of data that shows that depleting the gut microbiome has far-reaching effects (metaphorically and literally) on human health. The fact of the matter is that 80 percent of immunity resides in the gut. It is the gut microbiome that determines how human metabolism functions, how strong one's immunity is, how the central nervous system responds (via something called that gut-brain axis), how hormonal function is regularized—basically it determines how healthy an individual is. Ayurveda has recognized this and has been promulgating a strong causal relationship between the human diet and health for the past 5000 years at least. At long last, science has caught up with Ayurveda.

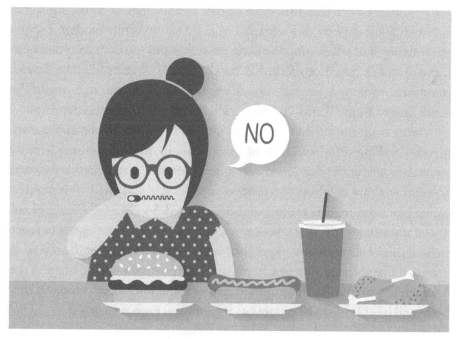

CHAPTER 6

A Streetcar Named Desire: The Role of Ayurveda in Reproductive Health, Childbirth and the Baby's Early Years

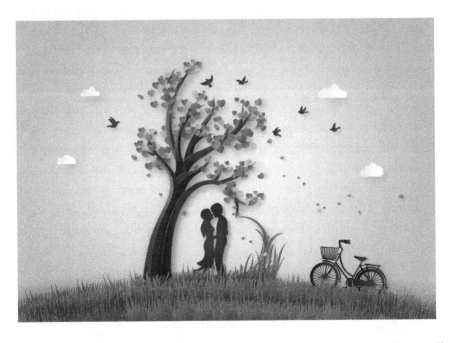

HIRAL SITS IN the doctor's waiting room, her foot jiggling nervously. She scrolls through her phone absent-mindedly, but every time the doctor's door opens and a patient leaves, her attention snaps to the display board showing the next ticket number.

She is at one of the best hospitals in her town, waiting for her follow-up appointment with a top-rated OB/GYN doctor. Hiral has valid reasons for feeling nervous. She has been in this very situation multiple times before—waiting in a doctor's sitting room, hoping for help. But to date, that necessary medical help hasn't come her way.

It all started when Hiral was about 15. Her menstrual cycle, which had never been that regular, to begin with, had started going absolutely haywire. She would miss her periods for a month or two, and then when it finally arrived, she would experience an unnaturally heavy cycle. This would leave her fatigued and in debilitating pain, often causing her to miss a few days of school. Concerned about the missed periods, her mother had taken her to a gynecologist. After a quick checkup, the doctor had told Hiral that menstrual cycles don't often regularize until one is much older. At her age, she had nothing to worry about. And as for the pain, well, that was just a normal part of having periods! Hiral had tried explaining that none of her other friends seemed to be having so much trouble, but the doctor had waved her off, saying that people usually had varied experiences.

A few years passed, and Hiral turned 18. But she was not the same cheery Hiral as before. Her cramps and the irregular cycle had proved to be quite disruptive to her teenage life. She would have to miss school every so often, which left her stressed out about her upcoming board exams. She had loved dancing, but she had had to miss several classes due to pain and fatigue. Her classical dance teacher had not taken kindly to that. Too embarrassed to explain the real reason for her frequent absences, she had eventually dropped out.

To make matters worse, Hiral had also started feeling extremely self-conscious about her looks—so much so that she had all but stopped going out with her friends. Her face was dotted with acne scars, and she was noticing a sudden surge of hair growth on her upper lip, chin, and arms. She definitely wasn't as thin as her friends either. At an age when teenage girls are most conscious about their appearance, these changes had not been great for her confidence levels. Her mother had tried gently coaxing her out of her shell saying, 'These are just hormonal changes—I'm sure many girls your age must be going through this. And what teenager doesn't get pimples?'

Her mother had taken her to a couple of other doctors over the years, but their response hadn't been too different from that first gynecologist all those years ago. She was just at that age. Irregular periods are nothing to worry about. Was she sure she wasn't exaggerating her pain? Had she tried losing some weight?

⊷⊶

Now, at 23, Hiral is in a much better place. Despite her health issues, she has managed to get into a great college. She has graduated with flying colors and landed her dream job as a legal consultant. And for the first time in her life, she has an inkling about what lay at the root of her menstrual inconsistencies. It is a condition that several of her friends and acquaintances suffered from—polycystic ovary syndrome or more commonly, PCOS. Their experiences had seemed eerily similar to her own, leading her to suspect she had it too.

That led her to explore more options and reach out to more specialists. Eventually, one gynecologist had referred her to an endocrinologist. An array of tests followed, but finally, here she was, for her follow-up appointment with the OB/GYN doctor.

The door swings open and another patient leaves. The display board finally shows Hiral's ticket number. She goes in. After reading her test reports and the endocrinologist's notes, the doctor confirms it. Hiral does indeed have PCOS.

And there it is! After almost a decade of being told her experiences were 'normal' and 'nothing to worry about,' she finally has a diagnosis. A name for what she has been going through. An actual disorder that was causing her all that pain, suffering, and anguish. Now that it has been identified, she can finally get some treatment.

'So, doctor, what next?' she asks eagerly.

'Are you planning to start a family soon?' the doctor queries.

'No,' Hiral replies. At just 23, she still has a lot to do before she gets married and has kids.

'Well, there's nothing you can do about it now. Come back when you want to conceive.'

Polycystic Ovary Syndrome

Hiral is just one of a large, large group of women going through this experience. Polycystic ovary syndrome is one of the most common disorders among women of reproductive age. In fact, it is so common that you probably already know several women suffering from PCOS—you might have already guessed the reason behind Hiral's experience, even before I revealed her diagnosis. Back in 2012, the World Health Organization (WHO) had put the global estimate of women affected by PCOS at 116 million. In India, it is estimated that the condition affects 10 percent of women[3]. That is a massive number in a population this large. However, given that identification is not quite so straightforward, we still don't have a lot of published data about this.

Polycystic ovary syndrome is an endocrine disorder that affects the development of eggs produced in the ovary and causes an imbalance of reproductive hormones. As the name suggests, the condition is characterized by multiple, fluid-filled cysts forming in the ovary, each containing an egg. However, these eggs never reach maturity and are never released through the process of ovulation. This, in turn, means the uterine lining is not shed—and this is what causes the irregularity in the menstrual cycle. Under normal circumstances, the ovaries produce estrogen and progesterone (the female hormones), and a small quantity of testosterone (the male hormone). But interrupted ovulation leads to exceptionally low levels of estrogen and progesterone, while the levels of testosterone are comparatively high. All these factors manifest in a wide variety of symptoms and fallouts.

---

3 https://www.sciencedirect.com/science/article/pii/S1110569016301510

- **Reproductive issues**. Interrupted egg maturity and the lack of proper ovulation lead to a lot of fertility issues. PCOS is one of the biggest causes of infertility amongst women. In women with PCOS, 70–80 percent have trouble conceiving, and even if they do, they face double the risk of premature delivery than women without the condition.[4] Chances of miscarriage and the risk of other gestational complications are also extremely high.

  A build-up of uterine lining over a long time can increase risks of endometrial cancer too. Should this happen, the patient might be sent in for an emergency hysterectomy, even at the peak of her childbearing years.

- **Metabolic ramifications.** Apart from reproductive functions, PCOS also has a huge impact on other metabolic activities. Between 60– 80 percent of women suffering from PCOS develop a resistance to insulin—a likelihood that jumps to 95 percent in women who are obese.[5] This is unfortunate because approximately 30 percent of PCOS patients are obese.[6] As most of us already know, obesity aggravates and exacerbates other diseases and disorders.

  A lot of women with PCOS (whether or not they are obese) are at the risk of developing cardiovascular disorders and high blood pressure. Diabetes is another major cause for concern. According to the Centers for Disease Control and Prevention (CDC), 50 percent of women suffering from PCOS stand to become diabetic or prediabetic, even before they turn 40.[7] They may also develop glucose intolerance.

---

4 https://www.healthline.com/health/polycystic-ovary-disease#pregnancy-and-pcos

5 E. K. Barthelmess and R.K. Naz, (2014), 'Polycystic ovary syndrome: current status and future perspective,' *Frontiers in Bioscience (Elite edition)*, *6*, 104–119, https://doi.org/10.2741/e695.

6 E.K. Barthelmess and R.K. Naz. (2014), 'Polycystic ovary syndrome: current status and future perspective,' *Frontiers in Bioscience (Elite edition)*, *6*, 104–119, https://doi.org/10.2741/e695.

7 'PCOS (Polycystic Ovary Syndrome) and Diabetes,' last modified March 24, 2020,

- **Psychological fallouts.** As if the physical fallouts were not grave enough, PCOS has been shown to have some pretty serious psychological impacts too. Hormonal imbalances are correlated with several mental health issues—anxiety and depression are very common amongst women suffering from PCOS. High levels of testosterone (hyperandrogenism) cause weight gain, excess hair growth, acne, and dark patches on the skin, so it often causes terrible body image issues and has a devastating impact on self-confidence. In a particularly vicious cycle, these factors only go on to heighten depression and other mental health issues that these women might be already suffering from.

Unfortunately, despite these severe consequences to physical and mental health, allopathic medicine is still unequipped to diagnose and treat polycystic ovary syndrome effectively. Many women report feeling dismissed, unheard, and unsupported by health care providers. Even though their symptoms may set in quite early on in puberty, they are often attributed to other causes, and the disorder is not diagnosed until several years have passed. One survey revealed that women have to consult over three medical professionals and it's almost two years before they get a diagnosis.

Even after diagnosis, there is a startling lack of information, and patients are often not guided through what they can expect and how they can manage their symptoms. Sometimes, birth control pills and drugs that regulate the levels of insulin in the body might be prescribed. However, these only work to manage the symptoms—they do not cure PCOS (allopathy currently does not have a cure for the disorder).

To Treat or Not to Treat—That's an Awful Question!

The worst-case scenario arises when PCOS is treated only as a reproductive disorder. Like in Hiral's case, many doctors only show due concern when

---

https://www.cdc.gov/diabetes/basics/pcos.html.

the woman in question wants to start planning for a baby. But this is not a safe route to take—and here's why. Although the symptoms of PCOS might become more evident during a woman's reproductive years, it is actually a chronic disorder that affects her throughout her lifespan. After all, comorbidities like diabetes and cardiovascular disease impact women even in their adolescence and post-menopausal years. It is also unfair and downright bizarre to expect them to bear the physical and psychological burden throughout their lives, except for the few short years when they actually want to conceive!

So, despite this, why do so many allopathic doctors continue to link the disorder only to reproduction? Of course, lack of awareness is one major issue. But one of the main reasons why doctors do this is because they are concerned about the cost-benefit ratio. Essentially, they think that the cost of taking the medicines available (we're talking about some terrible side effects here) far outweighs the benefits of taking them. That is, not until these women come to a point where they are making potentially life-altering decisions—of whether or not they want to have a baby.

Allopathic hormonal contraceptives are often prescribed to regulate and regularize the menstrual cycle. But these pills are notorious for having several very inconvenient side effects. Some women experience sudden weight gain—which is ironic since, as we have already seen above, being overweight aggravates many of the symptoms of PCOS. Others experience body pain, brutal migraine attacks, spots, and skin discoloration. Psychological side effects include horrible mood swings, which sometimes go so far as to cause long-lasting mental health issues (again, the irony!). One study of over a million women actually found that teenagers taking these pills were 80 percent more likely to develop depression.[8]

Drugs that regulate the levels of insulin in one's body, which are also commonly prescribed for PCOS, have been found to have unpleasant gas-

---

8 'The pill is linked to depression–and doctors can no longer ignore it,' last modified October 3 2016,
https://www.theguardian.com/commentisfree/2016/oct/03/pill-linked-depression-doctors-hormonal-contraceptives.

trointestinal side effects. Think nausea, vomiting, diarrhea, and loss of appetite. These drugs have also been linked to vitamin B12 deficiency (which has far-reaching effects like atrophic gastritis, fatigue, heart palpitations, digestive issues, memory loss, behavioral changes, and sometimes even depression) and an accumulation of lactic acid in one's blood. Pair these with the side effects of the hormonal birth control pills—and you might find yourself agreeing with the doctors who are hesitant to prescribe them.

The Ayurvedic Response

That is not to say that women who suffer from PCOS *and* do not fancy going about their day feeling bloated, nauseated, and depressed are doomed to a life of pain and uncertainty. Ayurveda doesn't just manage the symptoms—it offers a complete cure.

Ayurveda leverages something called phytohormones, which are plant materials that mimic or trigger hormonal activity in humans. You might already be familiar with the functionalities of plant hormones in your diet—you may know that a diet rich in gibberellic acid (think grains and spinach) can help reduce inflammation, while fruits and veggies like apricots, apples, and carrots (which are rich in the plant hormone abscisic acid) can help regulate and control certain aspects of diabetes.[9] Phytohormones are used in Ayurveda to treat and cure hormonal disorders, clear pelvic obstructions, and normalize one's metabolism—thereby helping in regulating the menstrual system.

Ayurvedic treatments for PCOS include the usage of plant materials like triphala kwatha, chandraprabha vati, and manibhadra choorna, which are great for clearing obstructions. Triphala also has the added benefit of being good for weight reduction. Shatavari, a kind of asparagus, helps balance and regulate the menstrual system, while krishna jeeraka oil (Nigella sativa) and the powdered form of a certain kind

---

9   Cell Press. 'How humans and their gut microbes may respond to plant hormones.' *ScienceDaily*, www.sciencedaily.com/releases/2017/08/170822123844.htm (accessed April 2, 2021).

of geranium (P. graveolens) are known to have properties that help destroy cysts and stimulate follicular maturity.[10]

Of course, Ayurveda never prescribes medicines in isolation, so a combination of yoga and pranayama are also usually recommended as a part of PCOS treatment. This further helps regulate the hormones and keep one's weight in check. The exact kind of yoga, pranayama, and other exercises are prescribed as per the individual's physiology.

I only got to know Hiral a few years after the events that opened this chapter. After years and years of physical and mental anguish, and having found no treatment for PCOS even after diagnosis, she was advised to seek Ayurvedic treatment by a friend. That's when she came to our practitioners. Again, she sat in a waiting room, nervously scrolling through her phone, dreaming about finding a solution, but not really holding out high hopes. But that's where the similarities with her previous experiences ended.

We were able to confirm her diagnosis and offer the correct treatment. Our practitioners prescribed a combination of the treatment described above. Ayurveda being the holistic form of treatment that it is, Hiral was also asked to make certain changes in her lifestyle and diet. Far from the dismissive suggestions of losing weight that she was used to getting from doctors, Hiral was pleasantly surprised to receive proper, step-by-step guidance. A few months down the line, she started noticing the changes. Her body mass index (BMI) was at a healthier level, and she felt like she had a lot more energy than before. For the first time in her life, she started noticing some semblance of regularity in her menstrual cycle.

Fast forward a few more months, and Hiral was able to come off her medication completely. The healthy diet plan (there it is again—a healthy diet!) and workout routine were all that she needed after that. Her cycle became completely regular—something that she had not dared to hope for before. She no longer had to worry about missed periods followed by

10 S.A. Dayani Siriwardene, , L.P. Karunathilaka, N.D. Kodituwakku, and Y.A. Karunarathne, (2010). 'Clinical efficacy of Ayurveda treatment regimen on Subfertility with Poly Cystic Ovarian Syndrome (PCOS),' *Ayu, 31*(1), 24–27. https://doi.org/10.4103/0974-8520.68203

sudden heavy cycles that would leave her bedridden for days. She no longer faced the risk of various comorbidities due to PCOS.

Reproduction

A few years later, Hiral decided she was ready to start a family. If she had followed the advice of the allopathic specialist, this is when a team of medical professionals would be scrambling to get her body ready for conception. She'd have been asked to go through innumerable tests and procedures (all super expensive, of course), which may or may not have succeeded. As it so happened, with the Ayurvedic treatment that Hiral had opted for, her system was already in a better shape than it had been in years. She was ready and prepped for this new step in her life!

And I am happy to report that Hiral was indeed able to conceive without much trouble or external intervention. She carried her baby to term and is now the mother of a healthy two-year-old girl. Hiral's story is just one of the many, many instances in which we were able to use the Ayurvedic approach to take care of not just a woman's reproductive desires, but her overall health and well-being too.

With that, let's now focus on reproduction and family planning. What about when a couple does want to start thinking of having children? What kinds of disorders, treatments, and lifestyle changes do we have to keep in mind then? Let's break it down into three phases—conception, pregnancy, and postpartum healthcare.

1. Conception

So far, we have discussed at length about PCOS and the ways in which it can hinder a woman's ability to conceive easily. Today, it remains one of the biggest causes of infertility. But of course, when it comes to conception, we have to look at both sides of the equation—the man and the woman.

Today, we see hundreds of fertility clinics spring up in every city in India, catering to both men and women. The in vitro fertilization (IVF) service vertical alone is expected to reach $775.9 million by the year 2022.[11]

---

11 https://www.franchiseindia.com/wellness/this-is-why-the-ivf-services-market-is-

Of course, there are many reasons that may be contributing to this sudden boom.

A woman who has no history of PCOS may still find it difficult to conceive because of various contributing factors. These include blockages in the fallopian tube, ovarian disorders, endometriosis, and even external factors like stress and poor lifestyle.

While the female reproductive system is understandably more complex, in about 40 percent of infertility cases, the reasons are traced to male factors.[12] And we're not just talking about erectile dysfunction either. Ayurveda identifies multiple doshas that can cause infertility among men.

- **Shukra dosha:** These are the most obvious biological factors that first come to mind. It basically means that the quality and quantity of the man's sperms are not optimal for conception. This covers everything from low sperm count, sperm movement, obstructions, and blockages among other things.
- **Aahara dosha:** This refers to improper food habits and improper digestion, which might not be giving the man the nutrients he needs.
- **Vihara dosha:** This covers all lifestyle-based factors that might be causing male infertility—lack of proper exercise, too much alcohol, drug use, and so on.
- **Manasa dosha.** Ayurveda does take mental factors into account while treating male infertility. Too much stress, mental exhaustion, inability to focus—all these can impact sperm quality or cause erectile dysfunction, leading to infertility.
- **Compromised bala:** This refers to the external physical factors that might be hindering a man's chances of fathering a child. For instance, certain diseases, weaknesses, past testicular trauma, or infections can be the reason for male infertility.

---

booming-in-india.13191

12 https://www.ncbi.nlm.nih.gov/pmc/articles/PMC6891995/

An Ayurvedic regimen can be a fantastic way to overcome fertility-related issues in a man as well. The holistic treatment would, of course, involve several lifestyle and dietary changes. He would be asked to follow a certain diet and prescribed a regular workout routine too. If he is found to be obese, the focus will be on weight loss—but even if his weight is not the issue here, a healthy diet will be prescribed to detoxify his system.

In stark contrast to all the synthetic 'wonder drugs' that claim to cure male infertility (leaving a variety of side effects in their wake), the Ayurvedic system falls back on a simple plant-based cure. Enter ashwagandha—a shrub that is native to India and Africa. The root of this shrub has been in use in Ayurvedic medicine for thousands of years.

There have been many studies conducted in recent years to test the effects of Ashwagandha on the sperm quality of men who have oligozoo-spermia, azoospermia, and various other inhibiting factors that prevent them from having children. The results of these studies confirmed what our ancestors already knew. Taking an extract of this root for just three months resulted in a significant increase in sperm count, motility, and semen volume. The root has various antioxidative and anti-inflammatory properties as well and has been found to lower cortisol levels. This helps tackle stress, inflammation, infections, and other secondary factors that might be contributing to fertility issues. Our practitioners recommend ashwagandha to be taken with a mixture of several other herbs for best results. And the best part is that it leaves no lasting side effects to be concerned about.

If the man and the woman both follow a regular diet and exercise plan and use the prescribed uterine tonics and supplements, their reproductive balance should be restored in a few months' time. And who knows—if enough people start seeing the wisdom in these ancient practices, maybe there will be no need for so many fertility and IVF clinics by the year 2022! (of course, I'm sure the folks who invested heavily in these fertility clinics will not be too happy about this)

2. During pregnancy

In movies, whenever there is a huge party or gathering and one particular woman refuses an alcoholic drink, that's our cue to know that she's pregnant!

Indeed, as per our modern lifestyle, pregnancy is usually linked to restrictions of various kinds, especially when it comes to the mother's diet. Most of us know right off the top of our head what an expecting mother should not have—alcohol, caffeine, sushi, seafood, and so on. But the 'dos' of a mother's diet during pregnancy are not as widely known beyond what our common sense already tells us. Of course, we know she should have fresh, healthy food with lots of fruits and veggies, and avoid processed foods as much as possible. But these are generic recommendations applicable to anyone—male or female, pregnant or not pregnant.

However, as important as what a mother does not eat during pregnancy are the things that she does eat. In the previous chapter, we discussed how most illnesses are a result of unwholesome dietary habits and a build-up of 'ama' due to improper digestion. This becomes especially true during pregnancy. Being born healthy is of utmost importance, as birth defects and complications can end up having far-reaching impacts on the child's life.

Ayurveda, thus, prescribes specific dietary guidelines for an expecting mother to ensure her health and the proper development of her child. These guidelines have less to do with restricting the mother's diet and more to do with supplementing it. Acknowledging the fact that different parts of the fetus develop in different stages of the pregnancy, these guidelines change on a month-on-month basis. Here's an overarching look at these guidelines:

Months 1 and 2: This is a very early stage of the pregnancy, and most people may not even realize that they are pregnant yet. It may take a month or more to confirm the pregnancy, depending on where the woman is in her menstrual cycle. However, this is also a precarious stage of the pregnancy, so once it is confirmed, the dietary guidelines work to stabilize the fetus and nurture the womb. It is recommended that the mother increases her consumption of light, cooling liquids at this time—think coconut water, juicy fruits, cool milk. Water chestnuts are considered to be a particularly 'garbhasthapan' food, which means it helps stabilize the fetus. So, early on in the pregnancy, a spoonful of powdered water chestnut is mixed with lukewarm milk and given regularly to the mother. And when I say milk, I mean A2 milk. Make sure you try to source this wherever you are. Nowadays, A2 milk is available in most places thanks to awareness and overall demand. Of course there are articles that say A1 milk and A2 milk are the same and that there is no difference between the two. Ignore such piffle. Let's be guided by Ayurveda and science. Not by agenda-driven articles!

Month 3: Milk is an important part of the mother's diet at this stage. It is recommended that she have lots of rice and milk, especially during the early meals of the day. Warm milk mixed with honey is also given as a soothing, comforting drink. Certain physicians also advocate the consumption of ground gooseberry rind. Specifically, have rice with milk (Boil with—one part rice, two parts milk, cow's ghee, mung dal, jaggery). This is recommended for breakfast and lunch.

Month 4: This is when the baby's body starts getting more defined, and sensory and motor functions start forming. This triggers certain cravings in the mother, and it is interesting to note that Ayurveda advises that unless these cravings go against any health conditions that the mother has, they be satisfied as much as reasonably possible. As far as general dietary practices go, wholesome foods like rice with curds and ghee (clarified butter) are recommended. Semolina halwa made with milk and jaggery or unrefined sugar is a good item to have that helps with the fetus heart development. You need to increase your food intake in the fourth month.

Month 5: The baby's mind starts developing in this phase, so foods that enhance mental faculties are recommended here. Again, cow's milk makes up an important part of the diet, along with rice and butter. When it comes to fruits, mangoes are considered especially nutritious, protecting the mother and baby from infections and diseases. Carrots, apples, and leafy greens are also recommended. A very specific jaggery and rice combination with four parts of rice, two parts of milk, one part ghee, one part jaggery and coconut (pieces) is extremely beneficial to the fetus. This is known as 'chakkara pongal' in South India and is made during the festival of Sankranti. Other foods to be taken during this month are one banana with dates per day. Figs and ghee every day is recommended for the health of the foetus. As far as fruits go, AVOID Morris bananas. Try to go for fruits that are grown locally and are indigenous to the area in which you live. As a thumb rule, bananas are NOT to be taken in combination with milk as this particular combination is not good for digestion.

Month 6: This is when the part of the brain that determines the baby's intellect and power of recollection develops. Ghee plays the starring role in the mother's diet here. One tablespoon pure honey in the morning after brushing teeth is very beneficial as per Ayurveda. The mother must eat curd rice. As per Ayurveda, the child's 'Medhas' (INTELLECT) will improve if the mother follows this particular diet.

Month 7: The baby's organs and features develop to a great extent in this month, and from this stage onwards, it is recommended that the mother's diet be determined as per her individual body constitution. This is also the stage when her stretching belly might start feeling uncomfortable and itchy, so her diet may include foods to alleviate this. Jujube berry infusions or medicated butter may be recommended. Turmeric rice (prepare rice with turmeric + pepper powder + cumin powder + salt as per taste) is to be taken once a day. Chandrashura seeds (watercress seeds) roasted in ghee and mixed with milk and sugar (again when I say sugar, I mean only the unrefined kind) helps in general debility and pregnancy-related anemia.

---

11. Food in Pregnancy- An Ayurvedic Overview; Vaidya R.M. Nanal; Anc Sci Life. 2008 Jul-Sep; 28(1): 30–32.

Months 8 and 9: This close to the delivery, the mother's diet starts becoming simpler, lighter, and more personalized. Rice gruel, certain diuretic herbs, and ghee-roasted watercress seeds are usually given to the mother at this time.

As you may have noticed, dairy products like milk, ghee, butter, and curds make frequent appearances in the dietary recommendations during pregnancy. I also recommend home-made paneer as a great source of healthy fat and protein. Fresh fruits and vegetables are, of course, endorsed too. However, milk and fruits are generally considered to be incompatible, so it is advised not to consume them together. Healthy fats like coconut oil, ghee, nuts, avocados, and seeds are instrumental in helping the mother put on enough pregnancy weight, and in developing the baby's brain.

Ayurveda recognizes that above all, the expecting mother should be kept happy and healthy (I wonder if this is why it is recommended that she spends most of her pregnancy with her parents rather than her husband). Particular kinds of exercises are advocated to keep her body fit, healthy, and well prepared for childbirth. Stress, anxiety, grief, and other negative emotions can affect the proper development of the embryo and can result in low birth weight. Sudden shocks and scares are obviously not good for pregnant mothers—in fact, some women report heightened senses during pregnancy, and they can find loud noises or disturbing images particularly distressing. The family, thus, plays a huge role in creating a warm, soothing environment for the expecting woman. Good food, soothing music, clean spaces, gentle aromas, harmonious living situations, and lots of rest are conducive to a happy, healthy pregnancy.

Here are some other general recommendations during pregnancy[11]:

1. Regular use of locally grown green leafy vegetables during pregnancy is recommended to prevent abortion and hemorrhage.
2. Apricots with honey are a very effective nerve tonic. It increases blood and cures constipation. It prevents infections and lowers the chances of degeneration of cells. It is a fruit rich in vitamin A

according to modern nutrition. Hence it is a very valuable fruit in the prevention of all the diseases caused by its deficiency.

3. Banana with dates, figs, and ghee every day in pregnancy is one of the best natural tonics. It also improves the blood picture during pregnancy and hence prevents pregnancy-related anemia to a great extent.

4. Milk and banana is not a healthy combination and it is best to avoid in pregnancy.

5. It tones up the large intestine, which helps in relieving constipation. Addition of fresh dates to the mixture gives good results for constipated mothers.

6. Dates—Soak four to six dates in fresh cow's milk overnight and grind the mixture next morning. This preparation with a pinch of cardamom powder and one teaspoon honey is used regularly to generate blood and bones of the growing baby.

7. Mangoes are very nutritious and preventive for frequent attacks of common infections like sinusitis, colds, etc. Drinking mango juice (Amra ras) with ghee and milk two times a day during pregnancy prevents fetal abnormalities. It increases the resistance of the fetus against infections, helps in proper development, eases delivery, and prevents post-partum complications.These are all, of course, general recommendations. The mother's pre-existing health condition must naturally be taken into account before following these guidelines. For example, if she is allergic to any of the foods mentioned above, then obviously that must be avoided. If she is particularly repulsed by a type of food for whatever reason, it makes no sense to stuff that down her throat just because it is recommended. As in all cases, common sense plays a very important role in observing these recommendations.

3. Postpartum care
For the mother

In a lot of countries, there is a good deal of focus placed on ensuring a happy and safe delivery. But the system breaks down when it comes to providing subsequent postpartum care and support to new mothers. Usually, mothers and babies are discharged from the hospital about two days after delivery, once the doctors have ascertained that they are in no need of any immediate medical assistance. After that, the new mother is expected to recover from the momentous experience her body has gone through *while* she is breastfeeding and taking care of a demanding new infant! That is a shocking amount of responsibility if you ask me. And if the mother happens to lack an adequate support system in the form of her family and partner, she is left to bear the burden on her own. Add to this the impossible standards set by the media—think of all those stick-thin celebrities photographed mere days after their delivery—and you'll see why so many new mothers feel overwhelmed by fatigue, stress, and depression.

Contrast this with the Ayurvedic system of postpartum care, which estimates 42 days as the ideal period required for healing after delivery. During these six weeks, it is understood that the mother's top priorities are to recuperate and bond with her baby. All the other necessities like looking after the baby and performing daily household chores are taken over by her support system—the members of her family or her midwife. Ancient Ayurvedic physicians like Sushruta, Charaka, and Kashyapa have all outlined detailed instructions for post-natal care, many of which are still widely followed today in India in many families. This includes:

- Receiving daily massages, either by a trained technician or a friend, followed by a warm bath and rest.
- Eating warm, fresh, preferably organic foods that are cooked well. The diet at this time usually consists of liquid-based, soupy dishes that are easily digested. It is recommended that the new mother have her heaviest meal at midday.
- Having small amounts of ghee (clarified butter) in the diet.
- Staying home and resting for three months before venturing out.
- Being in a warm environment free of drafts, dust, noise, and harsh lights.
- Avoiding overstimulation and engaging in quiet activity (this includes limiting TV time, especially at night).

- Limiting visits from friends and family to allow the new mother enough opportunities to rest and also to not expose the newborn to various germs (the baby's immune system is rudimentary at best during this stage).
- Receiving help with cooking, cleaning, shopping, and other chores. This, again, allows the new mother to rest and bond with her baby.
- Enjoying quiet meals, preferably with pleasant company.
- Breastfeeding (in fact, ideally this should be the only and main diet for the baby) and providing daily Ayurvedic massage for the baby.
- Practicing daily meditation.
- Maintaining an early bedtime (before 9:30 p.m.). This might seem laughable to hassled new mothers, but when you consider the traditional system of support that was available, this doesn't seem too unreasonable.

The process of childbirth is said to aggravate the 'vata' humor, so an Ayurvedic diet recommended to the mother at this time focuses on neutralizing this. She will be given a lot of warm, hearty soups, broths, and khichdis made with easy-to-digest vegetables and lentils. Healing spices like ginger, fenugreek, black pepper, and turmeric will be judiciously used. Dairy, again, plays an important role in this diet—some midwives actually administer up to two liters of whole milk to the recovering mother. Immediate weight loss is not expected from a new mom by any means. In stark contrast, she is given warm sweets, halwas, and laddoos made with wheat flour, urad dal flour, herbs, and lots of ghee and jaggery.

Apart from facilitating healing, postpartum nourishment has another important factor to keep in mind—that of boosting breast milk production. The Ayurvedic system recommends at least six to nine months of breastfeeding, which should be extended up to a year if possible. To ensure that the mother produces adequate quantity and quality of breast milk, she is given various herbs and plant-based supplements.

When you hear the term 'superfood,' you probably think of kale or avocados or chia seeds. But for a lactating mother, there's nothing better than shatavari. This is a kind of wild asparagus that grows in the Himalayan regions of India (it's very different from the asparagus that you find in your departmental stores). I call it a 'superfood' for good reason—it has so many curative properties and health benefits that Ayurvedic practitioners have recommended this to new mothers for centuries. In fact, even modern allopathic doctors prescribe this supplement as a common practice in India.

Shatavari is a galactagogue, which means it boosts the production of prolactin and corticoids, thereby enhancing the amount and quality of breastmilk the mother can produce. But that's not all it does. It has fantastic antioxidant and anti-inflammatory properties, which help prevent and repair cell damage—offering an amazing advantage for women who have recently gone through the physical stress of childbirth and are now experiencing exhaustion and lack of sleep. The herb also enhances the immune system, thereby helping the mother fight off infections and ensuring that she does not need extra medication while she is breastfeeding. Another great benefit? Some components in shatavari work as anti-depressants, which can be a boon for women experiencing post-baby blues.

For the baby

Some extreme naturalists will have you believe that the mother's breastmilk is all that a newborn baby needs. When it comes to nutrients and antibodies, that is certainly true—and that is why we do all we can to help the mother boost her breastmilk production.

But it is categorically untrue that the baby needs nothing beyond this. Proper vaccination is still very much required, and not following the recommended schedule can result in some very serious and far-reaching consequences for the child. As we have discussed in one of the previous chapters already, vaccination is certainly not a new concept or some kind of conspiracy. Ayurvedic physicians have been vaccinating and inoculating children for centuries, and it is definitely an age-old, tried, and tested practice. Even at our clinics, our physicians strongly recommend that new parents follow the vaccination schedule that is prescribed in the country they live in.

CHAPTER 7

Kapil Dev, an All-Rounder Par Excellence: The 360-Degree Holistic System that is Ayurveda

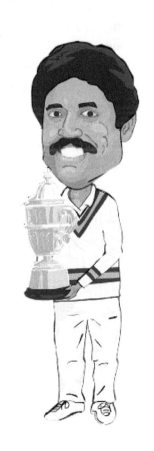

IT WAS THE summer of '83, and there was this feeling of desolation in the air. It was the cricket World Cup Finals, and India was all out with a meager 183 runs. Grim faces, angry mutters, and pessimistic predictions of doom and gloom filled our living room.

There are two things you should know at this point. First, in case you don't already know much about India's relationship with cricket, let me tell you that out here, it's not just a game. It is an obsession; it is the great unifier; it is almost the unofficial religion of India. So, when our team goes on to the World Cup Finals, most of us consider that a personal victory. And when we get bowled out at 183, we grieve like it's a personal loss.

Second, this particular World Cup Final against West Indies was held in 1983—a time when not every household had a television set. So, during momentous occasions and events like this, neighbors, friends, and family would congregate at the houses that did have a TV. Ours did, so we were playing host to a lot of people that day. With such a big crowd, the atmosphere tends to get particularly charged. I was 13 at the time, but I remember that day so vividly. Everyone was gathered around the TV—a lucky few had managed to snag chairs and stools, others were perched on any available surface, or sitting on the cool, red floor. My mom had rushed to whip up a huge batch of tea during the commercial break. It was being played in Lord's, the Mecca of cricket in England. With the time difference, it was beyond bedtime but we were super-charged with excitement and we wanted tea. "Tea, ma! We want tea with biscuits!" we pleaded. We were all clutching mismatched cups and saucers, eyes glued to the screen. That plate of biscuits sat untouched on the coffee table. As our last wicket fell, some people got up and left, too dejected to even watch the second innings. The rest of us persevered, but without much hope—we knew there would be no coming back from this. And we couldn't have been more wrong.

For in the second innings, one man stepped up and turned the match around. Kapil Dev, the Indian captain, ran faster than I thought was humanly possible and took a running catch with his back to the downward arc of the cricket ball (now for those who haven't played the game, let me tell you that to pull off this catch, you need to be supremely fit, have pin-point judgement, must be an excellent fielder, and possess nerves of steel) that would go down in history. Every single person there jumped up in unison, and the room absolutely erupted in cheers. I accidentally knocked over a cup of tea in my excitement, but even my mother was too elated to notice or care! We were so loud that the noise brought the neighbors—the ones who had walked away earlier—running back. That wicket was the turning point of the match. A few short hours later, India was lifting the World Cup. Kapil and his team had done it!

Thinking back, I don't know why we were so surprised. After all, Kapil Dev was known to pull miracles out of thin air. A couple of matches before this, he had proven his mettle as a batsman. India was playing against Zimbabwe and had already lost 5 wickets for just 17 runs. Kapil Dev walked out onto the pitch and single-handedly scored 175 runs, winning that match for us and helping India qualify for the next round.

Here's the thing about all-rounders—they can be depended upon. When things are looking down, you can count on them to step up and deal with the issue, whatever it may be. Do you see where I'm going with this?

Why We Need a 360-Degree System of Wellness

I strongly believe that when it comes to health care choices, we should all enjoy the benefits of a system that is an all-rounder. The Kapil Dev of health care, if you will. This is particularly important because many of us don't realize exactly how interconnected the different systems in our bodies are.

However, most of us have felt the effects of it from time to time—we have all noticed how certain triggers often affect systems that are apparently completely unrelated. For instance, you've probably seen how, when your digestive system is a bit off, you tend to feel cold. Or when you are going through some kind of emotional turmoil, your appetite takes a hit. And who here hasn't suffered a tension headache or broken out in pimples during times of stress?

But sometimes, these connections show through in unexpected ways. For example, some months back, I was at a family gathering. I was happy to catch up with my nephew, whom I hadn't seen since the previous year since he landed his first job at a big marketing and analytics firm. I was keen to know how he was enjoying his work life and newfound independence. He seemed passionate about the work and was clearly good at it too—he told me that on completing his first year at the firm, he had received a promotion. I congratulated him but soon realized that something was off. He was not as excited as I had imagined he'd be.

On probing, he told me that the new role would require him to relocate to Delhi—a city that has been touching record levels of air pollution over the last few years. He was so concerned that the pollution would aggravate his breathing problems, that he was thinking about turning down the promotion. Now, this may seem like a valid concern, except for one fact—I had never known my nephew to have a history of breathing issues.

Surprised, I asked him what he meant, and found out that he had been experiencing some difficulty in breathing over the last few months, especially at night. Although this wasn't confirmed by a doctor yet, he was scared that he was developing asthma. Over the course of our conversation, I got to know more about his job and new lifestyle—and it all seemed very hectic to me. I wondered if his breathing trouble at night might be a symptom of stress. He was surprised to hear this and brushed it off at first. After all, he liked his job. Sure, his role was challenging, but he enjoyed the challenge. I told him to think about it, and at least try some mindfulness tools or meditation, to begin with. He agreed, and sure enough, that seemed to go a long way in easing that shortness of breath he was experiencing.

We have touched upon the fact that Ayurveda is a holistic system a few times now. In this chapter, let's delve into what that really means. While a lot of medical systems treat symptoms individually, Ayurveda spots the links between them and treats them all together. Here are the major aspects of holistic Ayurvedic wellness.

1. **Physical health:** This refers to the internal as well as external aspects of the body. This covers everything from muscles, skin, and bones to the way your organs like the lungs, heart, and stom-

ach function. The signs and symptoms of any physical disorder, of course, are the easiest to track and treat.

2. **Mental and emotional health:** While mental health is a completely separate vertical in most medical systems, Ayurveda treats it as a part of the whole. It acknowledges the fact that a person cannot be considered 'healthy' as long as just their physical organs are working fine. If one is suffering from mental duress of any kind, it won't be long before it shows up as different symptoms in various parts of the body.

3. **Spiritual health:** Spirituality is not an easy concept to define, since it means different things to different people. Broadly, spirituality is the way one connects one's inner self to one's transcendent faith or belief system. Irrespective of what faith or belief system one follows, Ayurveda believes that spirituality plays an important role in overall health.

Thus, 'health,' when defined in Ayurvedic terms, encompasses the mind, body, and spirit. It ensures that all these aspects of one's self are functioning optimally and are in balance with one another.

The Three Tools of Holistic Wellness

Now that you know what Ayurvedic wellness aims to achieve, let us discuss how the system goes about achieving it. While most health care systems fall back on medicines when it comes to ensuring health, that is only the third pillar of holistic wellness in Ayurveda. There are two more pillars that come before it—diet and exercise. If the first two are done right, one would hardly ever need to resort to medicines to stay healthy.

In Chapter 5, we talked about Ayurvedic diets in great detail. We discussed how the perfect diet for you would be ascertained based on your body type and unique constitution. In this chapter, let's delve deeper into the concept of exercise.

When exercise and Ayurveda are mentioned together in the same breath, most people immediately think of yoga. And that's a reasonable thought process—yoga is, after all, an intrinsic part of Ayurvedic health and wellness. But the term 'exercise' in Ayurveda is much more than that. While we will talk about yoga in greater detail in the last chapter, here I would like to share some general Ayurvedic wellness techniques and tactics.

Physical fitness

Physical exercise is one of the most important pillars of Ayurvedic wellness. But don't take my word for it; take a look at what Sage Charaka said:

From physical exercises, one gets lightness, a capacity for work, firmness, tolerance of difficulties, elimination of impurities, and stimulation of digestion.

Sounds a lot like what a gym instructor would say when he's trying to get you to sign up for a year's worth of classes, right? But there's one crucial point where Charaka would have disagreed with modern gym instructors, and it is this. The modern concept of exercise seems to be all about pushing yourself.

'Don't stop till you drop,' says the motivational poster at your gym.

'No pain, no gain,' confirms your super buff friend.

'Sweat is just your fat crying,' claims a post from that fitness influencer you follow on Instagram.

Today, we are sold to this idea that pushing your boundaries is the right thing to do. And if you're not testing your limits—well, then you are just lazy. The other thing that modern fitness routines do is focus on numbers. What do you weigh? What is your heart rate? How many steps do you take per day? What should your calorie deficit be? Our obsession with numbers and stats has elevated the fitness wearables market to a whopping 50-billion-dollar industry.[13]

In stark contrast, Ayurveda goes by a concept that might seem radical in today's data-driven world—it tells you to listen to your body. It doesn't tell you how many kilometers you should jog or how many steps you should rack up. It does not promote extreme forms of workout or shame you for

---

13 https://codete.com/blog/wearable-fitness-technology-trends-and-statistics-2020/

not being intense enough. All it does is tell you that you should exercise regularly, and maintain a pace that feels steady and comfortable for you.

A far cry from pushing yourself beyond your limits, Ayurveda actually recommends that you only work out to half your capacity. And you don't need a smartwatch or a fitness tracker to tell you when you've reached this limit either—when you start breathing heavy and break out in a light sweat, that's when you know you're doing it right. Occasionally, it is fine to go beyond this too. If you're playing a sport that you enjoy and feel stimulated by, then keep playing by all means. But when your body tells you it has had enough, then go ahead and stop. After all, Ayurveda believes that exercise should bring you joy and fulfillment, not pain, tears, and exhaustion. (Enjoyment, again, is one aspect of exercise that is conspicuously absent from a lot of new workout routines!)

In the previous chapters, we've spoken at length about how, in Ayurveda, diet and medicine are highly customized as per the individual's unique constitution. Unsurprisingly, that is true for exercise too. Just like specific diets work well for some people but not others, so it is with exercise routines. An Ayurvedic practitioner may recommend a particular kind of workout to you, based on your dosha or dominant humor. Curious as to what these workout routines might look like?

- **Vata workouts.** It is understood that those with vata dominant body types have a hypermetabolic constitution, so they burn through their energy pretty quickly. So long-lasting endurance exercises are probably not going to be very enjoyable for these people.

  An Ayurvedic practitioner might suggest physical activities that are slow, fluid, and purposeful, with an emphasis on building strength. Think yoga, swimming, cycling, or exercises that focus on stretching and flexibility, rather than running marathons. This body type is also known to benefit from activities that are particularly grounded—so mat exercises or working out amidst nature might be recommended.

- **Pitta workouts.** Pitta dominant body types tend to have more stamina and endurance than vata dominant people, so moderate exercise is recommended with adequate periods of rest in between. It is understood that this category of people tends to be ambitious and willful, so they enjoy tasks that pose a challenge. However, these challenges need to be set keeping moderation and balance in mind.

  Pitta-specific workouts can include running, swimming, yoga, and dancing. Much like vata exercises, here too, the focus should be on grounding, fluidity, and stretching. Mat exercises, certain more fluid and vigorous forms of yoga, and nature hikes are good options.

- **Kapha workouts**. Those with this body type tend to be hypo-metabolic, so they are not likely to flash through all their energy reserves in one go. With their stamina, kapha dominant people enjoy more vigorous, enduring workouts. Long-distance running, hiking, aerobics, and endurance training might be recommended.

  However, on the flip side, kapha body types also have a tendency toward sluggishness and lethargy, so they might need more motivation to exercise at all in the first place. Having a single exercise routine every day will fast get monotonous and unexciting, so adding variety is essential to keep them engaged. Adventurous activities like hiking and climbing will likely work well when interspersed with endurance and strength-building routines.

Your preferences and choices are taken into account too. Ayurveda does not aim to keep you away from a sport or a workout that you enjoy if it just happens to go against your constitution. Instead, it aims to help you find a balance that will let you optimize your performance while keeping your body's needs in mind. So, for instance, if you happen to have a pitta dominant body type but also love to play a rigorous sport, an Ayurvedic practitioner will tell you what kind of rejuvenative practices you should embrace to ensure that your body heals well. You might soon find that playing the sport has become much more enjoyable, and you are performing better than ever before.

Mental wellness

To say that our modern lifestyle is hectic and fast-paced would be an understatement. Most of us reach for our phones as soon as we wake up, getting inundated in notifications and e-mails before we even get out of bed. And the day that follows often does not get any easier. The abundance of smart personal devices contributes towards an always-on lifestyle that keeps us tethered to work and obligations, no matter where we are or what time of the day it is. While working hard is certainly not a bad thing, being always-on is unsustainable at best. It is no surprise then that mental health issues like anxiety and depression are at an all-time high.

Although the ancient Ayurvedic physicians probably wouldn't have imagined a daily routine like ours today, they did see the importance of mental peace and wellness as a way to achieving holistic health. After all, certain emotions like grief, fear, and anxiety are timeless, and Ayurveda offers certain suggestions and recommendations to manage one's mental health that are more holistic.

For instance, for most people, stress manifests itself physically as digestive disorders. Acid reflux and heartburn are usually the first indications of stress that we experience. If you go to an allopathic doctor, they will prescribe medicines that will reduce the production of stomach acids. Alternatively, you might not go to a doctor at all and simply reach for your go-to antacids rather than working on managing your stress. However, these measures often prove counterintuitive—and lots of well-known acid and heartburn medications have been linked to graver health issues. Inhibited production of stomach acids, for example, can lead to the overgrowth of certain kinds of harmful gut bacteria—which contributes to liver inflammation and damage. A damaged liver, in turn, inhibits the production of certain enzymes, thus leading to issues like gastroesophageal reflux disease (GERD). Of course, this means you reach out for more antacids—and the cycle continues.

Other symptoms of stress include muscle spasms, panic attacks, trouble falling asleep, and so on. These, too, are treated with short-term solutions (think Valium, sleeping pills, etc.). Not only are they highly addictive, but they also have their own set of harmful side effects too, which trigger more vicious cycles of dependence.

In stark contrast, Ayurveda takes a more integrated approach through substances called adaptogens. These are materials that help the body deal with stress and fatigue in more natural and sustainable ways and have no harmful side effects. Ayurveda boasts of a vast repertoire of adaptogens like shatavari and ashwagandha. When combined in the right manner and prepared in very specific ways, they engage your hypothalamic, pituitary, and adrenal glands to enhance the production of the hormones that help you deal with stress. Adaptogens, thus, are extremely valuable for your psychological well-being.

Ayurveda also keeps in mind that stress responses work the other way round too—physical health often has mental consequences as well. For instance, the gut has a direct connection to the brain—physically through the vagus nerve, as well as chemically, through various hormones and neurotransmitters. Gut inflammation and imbalances in the intestinal microbiome can trigger anxiety, depression, and other mental health issues. Research has also revealed that this shows up in ways that actually resemble the symptoms of autism and Parkinson's disease in animals. Gut health, thus, is yet another thing that Ayurveda prioritizes when it comes to mental health treatments. This is nothing as simple as just taking probiotics—Ayurveda understands that the gut has to be suitably prepped to accept the 'good bacteria' that probiotics bring in. It thus also includes prebiotic supplements like triphala rasayanas and the like.

Triphala, which we have mentioned a couple of times already, is a formulation made of three plants called amalaki, vibhitaki, and haritaki, mixed in equal measures. It has a rich portfolio of therapeutic advantages—including dual benefits on gastrointestinal health and mental health. In fact, so taken was Charaka by this miracle mix, that he actually raved about it in his compendium—saying that triphala taken with honey and ghee can potentially help one live for a hundred disease-free years! Again, there are several methods of preparation of triphala. Different ratios of triphala are used to address different conditions. Many times, triphala is processed in specific decoctions to treat specific conditions. For examples, triphala triturated and levigated in decoctions of asana and lhadira one after the other is mandatory for patients with obesity and wanting to lose weight. In fact, it is said that a true Ayurvedic expert is one who knows how to use triphala in virtually all diseases states. Such experts are rare and this knowledge is very quickly getting extinguished. It is up to us to safeguard this for posterity.

Suggestions also include following a specific routine each day, and offer tips to enjoy quality sleep every night. Of course, following a diet and exercise plan as per your constitution makes up a big part of ensuring stability and overall wellness (as we discussed earlier, mental and physical health are intrinsically linked to one another).

Apart from this, Ayurveda also recommends various processes of purification and detoxification of the body. Concepts like 'oil pulling' and 'lymphatic drainage' might be trending now, with spas charging a hefty sum to provide these treatments—but they have been a part of the Ayurvedic method of detoxification for centuries now. The panchakarma method, for example, uses a combination of soothing oil massages, steam therapy, nasal oil treatments, lymphatic massages, and herbal enemas to get rid of toxins from the body.

Spiritual wellness

Here's a quick question. When someone asks you who you are, what do you tell them?

Most people answer using their jobs or relationships as reference points—'I'm a doctor,' 'I am a teacher,' 'I am a wife and mother,' and so on. And it makes sense. After all, if you're having a conversation at a party, you're hardly going to bare your soul to someone you've just met. But here's the thing—if you ask yourself the same question within the privacy of your own mind, is your answer going to be any different?

Today, most of us are so caught up with work, family, and other obligations, that those pretty much become our identity. Our busy lives mean that we barely have any time to check all the boxes off our to-do list, let alone take some time out to look inwards and reflect. However, that's just what Ayurveda suggests you do. Spiritual wellness is as important in Ayurveda as being physically and mentally fit. As I mentioned earlier, the concept of nourishing one's soul may seem pretty abstract and ambiguous today. But following an Ayurvedic wellness routine means we make space for a bit of soul-searching and spend a bit of time each day pursuing the goals of self-reflection and self-awareness.

Practices like meditation are thus extremely significant. Although Ayurveda does have its roots in the Hindu religious system, when it comes to meditation, it does not require one to only use Hindu chants and rituals. It welcomes you to meditate based on your own learnings and beliefs. While meditation might mean prayer to some people, for others it might mean finding a deep connection with oneself or with nature. And they are both perfectly fine.

Although Ayurveda does recognize that meditation might mean different things to different people, it does recommend some specific techniques and dos and don'ts. For instance, irrespective of what your beliefs are, if you're trying to meditate in the middle of a loud, crowded party, you're probably not going to be too successful. The dos, then, would include finding a quiet, peaceful place, grounding yourself with your spine erect, and closing your eyes. Many Ayurvedic meditation techniques start with breathing exercises, where you consciously focus on your own breath as you inhale and exhale. Awareness of one's own body is also a good starting point—several techniques recommend you follow your breath as it goes through your system. When you first start meditating, you might find your attention wandering, but this is entirely normal, and it gets easier to focus over time. In fact, those well-versed in the art of meditation claim that they often lose track of time as they sit in deep meditation.

Now Put Them All Together!

So far, I have discussed physical, mental, and spiritual health separately in order to introduce the Ayurvedic philosophy behind them. However, in more day-to-day, realistic practice, there is, of course, quite a bit of overlap between these three aspects of wellness. After all, massages are good for the body *and* the mind; meditation is also a great tool to ensure mental health; playing a sport is a fantastic way to stay engaged both physically and mentally.

So now, let's have a look at a couple of Ayurvedic wellness techniques that look after your body, mind, and spirit all together.

Surya Namaskar

Today, there are many conversations around the importance of wellness, self-care, and self-love. You read so much about how it is so important to find the time to work out, to reflect, to practice gratitude, and to give yourself a mental break. But add up the amount of time it takes to exercise, meditate, journal, and pamper yourself in the morning—and it may seem quite unachievable if you happen to lead a busy life. So, do you push those wellness practices to your weekends (and hope that you have enough time then) or do you try to pack them into your hectic morning hours, come what may?

Surya Namaskar is the perfect answer to this modern dilemma—it can help you bring those few moments of serenity and stability to your mornings. Surya Namaskar essentially means 'sun salutation.' Most ancient civilizations around the world had one thing in common — they all understood the life-sustaining power of the sun. The Surya Namaskar is a meaningful way to bring that ancient tradition back into your life by acknowledging and honoring the power of the sun. It is practiced by following twelve dynamic yoga poses or asanas in a particular sequence as your first activity every morning. It is usually practiced on an empty stomach.

But Surya Namaskar is not just a tool for practicing spirituality and gratitude. It has so many benefits and addresses so many physical concerns that any modern workout routine would be hard-pressed to match up to it. Here's a look at what it can do:

- **It is a great cardio workout**. It gives your body a fantastic workout, especially if you are looking to lose weight. Just 10 minutes of practicing the Surya Namaskar burns more calories than an equal amount of time spent swimming.
- **It strengthens and tones many different parts of your body**. Done right, you should be feeling the effects of these asanas in your abs, thighs, butt, and arms. Besides, it improves flexibility and limbers up your joints.
- **It improves various systems in your body.** Practicing Surya Namaskar regularly boosts the digestive system, circulatory system, and respiratory system among others.
- **It helps regularize menstrual cycles.** These asanas have a balancing effect on your hormones, which as we have seen in the previous chapter, is so important in regularizing periods.
- **It makes you glow.** Given that this sequence improves blood circulation and helps you absorb nutrients from your food better, it has a visible effect on your skin and hair. We're talking a real 'I Woke Up Like This' glow!
- **It relaxes your mind and helps you focus.** The positive effects on your mental health are no less astounding than the physical benefits. These asanas are challenging enough that they keep your mind engaged, while the deep breathing techniques that accompany the poses help you relax and clear your mind. The effects of this last through the day, and you may be surprised to find yourself calmer, more focused, and definitely more at peace.
- **It tackles insomnia**. Those who have trouble falling asleep at night swear by the benefits of this sequence. It helps relax your nerves and your emotions, which has a calming effect overall, and helps you drift off more easily.

Pranayama

When it comes to Ayurvedic wellness, there's one more ancient technique that has gained traction all over the world, and that is pranayama. 'Prana' refers to one's vital energy or life force. And there's nothing that enables that continued life force more than our breath. Pranayama, thus, is the science of controlling and regulating your breathing patterns.

Now, you might be familiar with a variety of breathing exercises—you might even use some of them as you practice yoga or mindfulness. But pranayama is more than just the act of regularizing your breath. It is the technique of conscious inhalation, breath retention, and exhalation following particular counts or maintaining certain intervals. There are various kinds of pranayama techniques, each prescribing a different breathing pattern and interval.

Pranayama is, as you may well imagine, a fantastic way to calm your mind and engage your spirit. But you'd be surprised at the sheer number of physical health benefits you can enjoy, simply by controlling and regulating your breath. To start with, it helps enhance your lung capacity, enabling you to take in fuller and deeper breaths each time. This automatically reduces stress and tension and helps you focus better. Apart from this, pranayama can also help lower cholesterol and blood pressure, thereby having a direct, positive impact on your cardiovascular health. More rigorous forms of pranayama can also help strengthen your stomach muscles, chest muscles, and diaphragm.

Describing all the different kinds of pranayama will make for a very extensive read—but let me share one particular pranayama exercise that I feel is very relevant in today's world. Given that hypertension is one of the most common lifestyle-led ailments today, this exercise comes in handy.

Here's a step-by-step guide to one form of pranayama that has been immensely beneficial in reducing hypertension—the count of eight is sacrosanct for this one:

1. Close your right nostril and inhale with the left nostril to the count of eight (for pace, think one Mississippi, two Mississippi, and so on, just like you were taught when you were young).
2. After inhalation, close your left nostril as well and hold your breath for 16 counts, keeping up the same counting pace.
3. Now exhale through the right nostril to a count of eight.
4. Now repeat the process by inhaling through your right nostril and exhaling through the left nostril. That completes one cycle.
5. Repeat the whole cycle eight times.

Sounds easy? Well, you may be in for a surprise once you actually start the exercise. You may notice that Steps 1 and 2 (inhalation and holding your breath) are easy, but the exhalation bit may start getting away from you. That's fine—you'll get the hang of it. Just try to finish exhaling at the count of eight exactly.

This needs to be done twice a day, over three months. Try doing the exercise on an empty stomach—before breakfast in the morning, and a few hours (three hours at least) after a heavy meal (your lunch presumably) in the evening. Three months down the line, you'll see noticeable improvements—you will likely not even need any further medication to keep your blood pressure in check! Well, that's not just the only benefit of pranayama. Here's something that might blow your minds off. Serious practitioners of pranayama have been found to live longer. Okay as anecdotes go—this seems all so fantastic and unbelievable and can be written off as coincidence. But is it really? Let me attempt to tease apart the science behind this and explain to you why this is from a cell biology and biochemistry perspective. First some basic biochemistry—all chromosomes of all vertebrates have structures at their very terminal ends called telomeres. Telomeres are DNA-protein complexes that protect the ends of the chromosomes from degradation or fusion or other DNA-repair processes. As we age, these telomeres keep getting shortened and indeed, telomere shortening has been hypothesized to be an age-related marker and age-related morbidity. Therefore, the balance of telomere-length control pathways dictates telomere stability. Under normal conditions, unstable telomeres have been associated with various disease states including diabetes, obesity, heart disease, chronic obstructive pulmonary disease, asthma, cancer, as well as psychiatric illnesses such as depression, anxiety, PTSD, bipolar disorder, and schizophrenia. Yoga and pranayama have been shown to have a positive effect on telomere length and stability. In fact, there is growing evidence that regular practice of asanas (yoga poses), pranayama and meditation (ALL integral aspects of Ayurveda) stabilizes telomeres. It is therefore not surprising to me at all that pranayama and long-time mindfulness practitioners live healthier and longer lives.

Chapter 8

Beauty is Not Skin Deep: Beauty Regimens in Ayurveda versus Cosmetic Cover-Ups

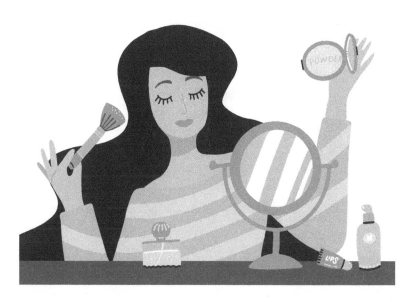

WHAT IS THE most bizarre my-life-is-a-lie moment you've ever experienced at a grocery store? Let me tell you mine.

Some years back, I was at a supermarket picking up some groceries. It was Friday, and I had invited some friends over to my house for lunch on Sunday, promising to cook my all-time brilliant palak paneer for them. I did my round of the store that Friday night, filled my cart with the things

I needed, and then came to the checkout queue. There were about three or four people with their carts full before me, so I knew it would be a while before it was my turn. Bored, I started looking around and my gaze drifted to the display cases of candies and chocolates and those mini-samosas they usually have near the checkout counter. That's when something caught my attention, and I did a double take.

There, on the display case, were rows and rows of chewing gum. One brand apparently had come up with a new variation and was given pride of the place next to the till. Bright posters and standees advertised the new flavor in big, bold letters—it was an Ayurvedic chewing gum!

Now, knowing a thing or two about Ayurveda, that claim struck me as extremely weird. Intrigued, I grabbed a pack to have a look at the ingredients. The gum was flavored with mint and neem oil, and those ingredients made up an understandably low percentage of the product. That's it— apparently, that's all it takes to market something as 'Ayurvedic!'

Such unscrupulous marketing practices are all around us these days. It feels like every other product in the market (detergents, creams, powders, toothpaste, you name it) are sold with a label that says 'Natural' or 'Herbal.' Some products don't even bother to make that claim—they put enough green on the label and let the consumers' assumptions do the rest. Well, fair play to them for such a savvy marketing trick, but what if you are one of the consumers falling for it?

In this chapter, I want to talk about the one industry that frequently employs these marketing tactics—the beauty and cosmetics industry. How do you spot such fake claims, what do they do to your skin, and what are the cleaner alternatives available? Let's explore.

The Clean Beauty Conundrum

Although many cynics will blame social media and celebrity culture for our fascination with beauty, our need to look good and be admired is certainly not unique to modern times. Though the idea of beauty has changed, humans have always looked for ways to enhance and highlight different features of their bodies. Ancient civilizations used fruits, flowers, and other natural products for this purpose. As society evolved, people found newer ways to enhance their beauty—often preferring to use harmful substances like lead paint on their faces rather than go natural. While modern beauty and makeup products have come a long way from that, they still cannot be considered strictly 'safe.' And consumers have started wising up to this fact.

Over the last few years, consumers are shifting to an overall more natural, sustainable lifestyle. They are extremely conscious about what they eat, what they wear, and what products they use in their homes. And they want their cosmetics, skincare, and haircare products to reflect these values too. Cue the popular new movement we know as 'clean beauty.'

Clean beauty embraces and promotes the use of products that are natural, sustainable, and non-toxic. Sounds fantastic, right?

While the concept of clean beauty is one that is much needed today, the reality is not quite so straightforward. Most countries don't regulate the beauty and cosmetic industry as strictly as one might imagine—and there is no watertight legislation by a governing body or even a clear definition when it comes to labels like 'clean,' 'safe,' or 'green.' That really means the term 'clean beauty' is open to interpretation. While some brands may mean non-toxic, another may mean sustainably sourced when they say their products are clean.

Now, you might not be too worried yet. 'That's fine,' you might be thinking. 'Rather than blindly trusting tags like clean or natural, I'll just turn the jar around and look at the list of ingredients.'

Well, that might not tell you much either. Remember the natural versus chemical debate we discussed in a previous chapter? Here's a quick recap:

- Everything, even harmless substances like water, has a chemical name
- Some chemicals are safe, while some natural substances are harmful
- Everything is safe or harmful in different doses

So, the long, complex, chemical-sounding ingredients listed on the label of your favorite beauty product may not mean much to you unless you have a degree in chemistry. Do also remember that different chemicals have completely different properties when used as different compounds. For example, propylene glycol is an ingredient that has been found to irritate the skin based on the amount that is used. So, if you have sensitive skin, you may not want this in your jar of face cream. The closely named dipropylene glycol, on the other hand, is commonly used as a solvent in many cosmetic products and is largely a safe ingredient. Not easy to remember, is it? Likewise, not all manufacturers and skincare experts agree on exactly how harmful or harmless a particular chemical is, and what are the safe quantities.

However, if you do want to be more mindful of what ingredients you should avoid, don't simply go by a label that says 'All Natural' or 'Chemical Free.' Here's a handy cheat sheet to tell you exactly which ingredients to look out for.

Reading Labels 101

1. **Parabens:** You may know about this one already since the harmful effects of parabens have been in the spotlight over the last few years. Parabens inhibit the growth of microorganisms, so they are commonly used as preservatives in shampoos, creams, and deodorants. However, parabens have been found to cause hormone imbalances that result in high levels of estrogen (the female hormone) in the body. And although this is still under debate, parabens have also been linked to tumors.

   May be listed as: -paraben, ethyl- or methyl-.
2. **Sodium lauryl sulfate:** You've probably heard of this one too—it's commonly referred to as SLS and is the ingredient that helps shampoos and body washes to foam up when you use them. However, SLS is a pretty harsh chemical that causes skin irritation, dryness, and redness, and can trigger allergic reactions.

May be listed as: sodium lauryl sulfate, sodium dodecyl sulfate, or simply SLS.

3. **Petrolatum:** Ever used a cream or a moisturizer that never seemed to get absorbed, and just stayed on the surface, making your skin look greasy? That may be petrolatum at play. Petrolatum often creates a barrier that prevents your skin from absorbing moisture. This means the ingredient actually dries out your skin from within while seeming oily or creamy on the surface.

May be listed as: mineral oil, benzene, paraffin wax.

4. **Formaldehyde:** This is used as a preservative (you may remember this from your high school biology lab, where it was used to preserve dead animal specimens). Unsurprisingly, it is not great for living human skin either. It has been linked to neurotoxins, scalp burns, hair fall, and may also be carcinogenic.

May be listed as: formaldehyde, formalin, glyoxal, bromopol.

5. **Phthalates:** This is the ingredient that makes cosmetics soft and easily spreadable. It also helps the product retain its fragrance. But phthalates may trigger hormonal disruptions in boys and young men, causing developmental and reproductive issues. It has also been linked to issues like diabetes and attention deficit hyperactivity disorder (ADHD).

May be listed as: phthalate, DBP, DEHP or DEP. More deviously, it is often listed simply as 'fragrance.'

6. **Hydroquinone:** If you have ever used a skin-lightening product, this may have been one of the ingredients listed there. Hydroquinone attacks the melanocytes, which is what gives your skin its pigment. However, as you may have guessed, this is a particularly harsh chemical, often causing your skin to look dull, blemished, or withered.

May be listed as: hydroquinone, tocopheryl acetate.

7. **Triclosan:** This chemical acts as an antibacterial ingredient, and is usually found in soaps, toothpaste, and deodorants. It also acts as a preservative and is commonly used to increase the shelf life

of cosmetic products. Triclosan is known to irritate the skin and trigger allergic reactions. A graver concern is that it can cause hormonal disruptions in the body.

May be listed as: triclosan (TSC) or triclocarban (TCC).

8. **Toluene:** You may know that pregnant women are often told not to color their hair. Toluene is one of the harmful ingredients responsible for this warning. This is a solvent that is often found in dyes and nail polishes. However, it is not good for you, even if you are not pregnant. Apart from causing birth defects, toluene has harmful effects on one's immune system and has even been linked to cancers.

May be listed as: benzene, methylbenzene, toluol or phenylmethane.

9. **Coal tar:** If you have a particularly bright lipstick or a vivid palette of eye shadow colors, check the ingredient list for coal tar. Coal tar is a viscous substance that is used as a base for bright, pigmented products. But it weighs heavy on your skin, often causing rashes, pimples, and acne. Coal tar is also known to have carcinogenic properties.

May be listed as: Artificial colors (like D&C Red #22, D&C Orange #5, and so on).

10. **Polyethylene glycol:** This is another ingredient that is commonly used in creams and thick lotions—but it triggers your sebaceous glands, causing your skin to produce excess oil. This can often lead to your skin breaking out in pimples and acne. It has also been linked to cancers and respiratory issues.

May be listed as: PEG (often followed by numbers).

Do note that the way you react to these ingredients will depend on a variety of factors—your skin sensitivity, the quantity of ingredients used, their percentage by weight, and so on. If this has put you off checking another ingredient label, I don't blame you. Standing in a poorly lit supermarket aisle going through an unpronounceable list of chemical components (printed in the tiniest font imaginable!) is not my idea of a good shopping expedition either.

A Safer Alternative

So, what do you do, given that you may not always be able to trust labels and you may not want to spend hours straining your eyes researching every ingredient that goes into your cosmetics?

Well, there is a safer alternative in Ayurveda. How exactly are Ayurvedic beauty treatments safer and better? Let's break it down.

1. **Natural:** As you may imagine, when it comes to providing solutions for skin and hair concerns, Ayurveda turns to natural ingredients obtained from plant and mineral sources. But given that we just finished talking about how 'natural' might not mean much on its own, let's explore this in detail.

    Let's come back to parabens for a minute. Did you know that parabens are derived from certain acids that occur naturally and organically? Particular kinds of berries, vanilla, and even vegetables like onions, carrots, and cucumbers are thought to contain these parabens. This prompts many cosmetic manufacturers to argue that they are entirely safe—after all, we eat these fruits and vegetables without any fallouts, right? But as we know, not everything natural is always safe. Moreover, when we ingest something, our digestive system metabolizes it in a way that is wholly different from the process in which it gets absorbed into the body when we apply it to our skin. So, it is a fallacy to say that just because one is safe, the other would be too.

    Hence, it is not enough to have natural ingredients in your cosmetic products—it must also be ensured that they are the *right* kind of natural. Ayurvedic haircare, skincare, and cosmetic products contain plant and fruit extracts that have been safely used by humans for thousands of years. Aloe vera, turmeric, honey, bhringaraj, and mulaithi are just some of the plant-based and natural ingredients that have historically been used to look after the skin and hair.

    When it comes to shelf life, it is not necessary to depend on chemical and synthetic preservatives either. A lot of people go by the thumb rule that if a product has a long shelf life, it indicates that it is full of chemicals—and subsequently, if a product is all-natural, that just means it won't last as long. While this is usually true, it is not absolute. It is quite possible to use natural preservatives to give you a long shelf life without you needing to worry about alarming side effects. Given that Ayurvedic beauty products usually utilize herbs, plant extracts, and milk as ingredients, they do frequently use these natural (read: safer) preservatives to keep the products fresh longer.

2. **Better absorption:** Skincare products that remain on the surface of your skin might not really give you too many benefits, irrespective of what they claim. They often end up forming a barrier that not only prevents your skin from absorbing moisture but also hampers its ability to expel toxins. This, in turn, can make your skin look dull and lifeless, and can trigger a lot of acne and pimples.

   The natural ingredients used in Ayurvedic cosmetic products have several biologically active components like peptides, vitamins, and antioxidants. This means that they get absorbed into the skin easily, and act from within. Not only does this make them more effective, but it also means that you might be able to use a lesser quantity of the product and still see a positive difference.

3. **Variety of benefits:** Plant and vegetable extracts and spices tend to be pretty versatile, with a single ingredient giving you a variety of advantages. Sandalwood, for instance, is one popular skincare ingredient that has been used in India for thousands of years. It is known to have antiseptic, antibiotic, anti-inflammatory, anti-aging, and hydrating properties. It protects the skin against sun damage and has a soothing effect if the skin is irritated by external pollutants. Plus, it has a gentle fragrance that eases stress and soothes anxiety—talk about a holistic approach!

   And that's just one ingredient. Likewise, Ayurvedic cosmetics make optimum use of many such powerful components that have multiple benefits. With one ingredient performing a variety of functions, you can get away with using fewer products on your skin. Not only is this way more cost-effective (most brands will try to get you to buy a separate product for each function!), it also means that your everyday routine is overall gentler on your skin—rather than layering quite so many products, you can just let your skin breathe.

4. **No side effects:** As you might already know by now, products and ingredients that have a multitude of side effects are not considered to be very good as per Ayurvedic terms. A shampoo that treats your dandruff but causes hormonal imbalance? A cream that smells good but puts you at risk for diabetes or reproductive disorders? These are bizarre trade-offs as far as Ayurveda is concerned.

Natural Ayurvedic cosmetics let you tackle all your skin and hair concerns and enjoy the benefits without having to worry about how they're going to impact your health over the long term. However, do ensure that you get your cosmetics from a trusted brand or source. As we have seen earlier, a few drops of herbal extract added to a heavily synthetic, chemical base does not make the product Ayurvedic. Such products might still end up causing all kinds of problems and side effects. When you choose a particular cosmetic, make sure it is as close to 100 percent natural as possible. This is especially true of products that you plan to put on the sensitive skin on your face.

5. **Bespoke:** Saving the best for the last—Ayurvedic cosmetic and personal care solutions can be customized according to your needs. When it comes to skin and scalp treatments, you may need to visit a practitioner who will recommend solutions based on your dosha. But even your everyday skincare products like cleansers, toners, and moisturizing oils and creams can be recommended based on your skin type. These solutions would also cater to those who have a combination of two doshas influencing their skin type. Of course, Ayurveda does also recommend switching up your skin and haircare practices

keeping your environment, lifestyle, and seasonal changes in mind.

But the customization goes much beyond this. Given that some treatments and solutions are not mass-produced, but are whipped up based on individual needs, Ayurveda is able to offer a more personalized approach to your beauty routine. We will discuss one example of this kind of bespoke solution later in this chapter.

The Fairness Unfairness

Growing up, sitting around in front of the television was not really the culture in my house. My brother and I were strongly encouraged to read, draw, or go outside to play. Not that we were complaining—we had a beautiful garden with five different types of mango trees, and many a happy summer evening was spent monkeying around with our equally boisterous bunch of cousins. But once we were older, we did sometimes enjoy a movie or some special show that was being broadcast that day. And we were equally fascinated with the advertisements—for chocolates, sodas, cosmetics, and shampoos. The ad for one particular product, however, sat uncomfortably with me even back then. It would always go like this.

A woman wants to be a TV anchor/ model/ dancer/ lawyer (really, just insert any profession that puts her in the public eye). Despite being the most talented person there, she doesn't make the cut. As she walks away dejected, she just knows that it is her dark skin that's holding her back (sometimes, her misgivings are confirmed—she overhears some snide jibes about her complexion as she walks away). Back at home, her loved ones tell her to take destiny into her own hands. Cue, that prized tube of skin-lightening cream. She applies it for a few days, and voila! She is fairer, happier, and suddenly oozing with confidence and self-worth. She decides to go back for that job interview, and this time, nobody can take their eyes off her. She is hired on the spot.

Unfortunately, in a lot of Asian societies, beauty is still equated with fairness. Skin-lightening lotions and creams make up a $450 million[14] industry

---

14 https://www.ncbi.nlm.nih.gov/pmc/articles/PMC5787082/#B2

in India alone, and dark-skinned people (especially women) are still habitually told to apply these products if they want to be considered good-looking. Wildly popular actors and actresses endorse these products, while magazines casually 'touch-up' photos of dark-skinned celebrities, lightening their complexion by several shades. Getting tanned is a big no-no, and beauty salons still recommend bleaching treatments to their duskier clients, even if they have just gone in for a cut and blow-dry!

In fact, in a recent controversy in India, brands that sell skin-lightening products were called out for continuing to propagate these racist and colorist stereotypes. Finally, in early 2020 the Indian Ministry of Health banned the promotion of these products. The manufacturers responded by simply dropping the word 'fair,' and continuing to sell the products under a more ambiguous name.

However, the Ayurvedic concept of beauty has nothing to do with fairness. It acknowledges the beauty in each person and encourages the acceptance of one's own unique skin tone. The harsh chemicals in skin-lightening creams are rightly recognized as extremely harmful, and no legitimate Ayurvedic range will offer such solutions. Beauty in Ayurveda, rather, has more to do with health and wellness—that particular glow of healthy skin, the shine and gloss of well-nourished hair, the sparkle in one's eyes when one is happy, fulfilled, and satisfied. Ayurvedic beauty products aim to make these available to everyone, irrespective of what color their skin is.

Ayurvedic Regimens

Ayurveda understands the importance of following a good beauty and grooming regimen irrespective of gender. For a lot of people, a morning routine is synonymous with getting ready for the day through external beautification—choosing one's clothes, doing one's hair, or applying makeup.

With an Ayurvedic morning routine, however, the focus shifts to holistic beauty. It may look something like this:

- **Waking up early:** Ayurveda recommends an early start for most people, though the exact time you wake up might be determined by your dosha.
- **Cleansing:** This involves splashing water on your face, and rinsing out your mouth and eyes. Some practitioners may recommend certain eyewashes, based on your dosha. Concepts like tongue scraping, gum massaging, and oil pulling have only started trending in Western countries recently, but these have been a part of Ayurvedic grooming routines for centuries now.
- **Detox:** This includes drinking a glass of warm water (some people prefer squeezing some lemon in it) to flush out the toxins in one's body. Administering ear drops, nasal drops, and clearing one's bowels are also a part of this step.
- **Exercise:** We have discussed the concepts of pranayama, Surya Namaskar, and meditation in detail in the previous chapter. These practices get your heart pumping and your blood flowing while also engaging your mind and your spirit.
- **Daily ablutions:** This refers to much more than just a shower. Ayurveda doesn't limit massages to the occasional spa visit—it recommends massaging your body with warm oil every day, in firm, repetitive motions. Not only does this nourish the skin, improve blood circulation, and promote better functioning of your internal organs, it also facilitates better lymphatic drainage (another concept that has gone mainstream recently). Gentle exfoliation—wet or dry—may also be practiced in this step.

Note the conspicuous absence of utilizing cosmetic cover-ups or skin-lightening masks! So, what should you do if you have spots, marks, or pigmentation that you want to get rid of? Here's where your Ayurvedic creams, lotions, and other beauty treatments come in. Wondering how these treatments work, if not superficially?

They work by improving circulation

Remember that glow I referred to earlier, which comes from having healthy skin? This is where I introduce the closest thing to a 'miracle potion' that we have in Ayurvedic skincare—kumkumadi tailam/serum. Kumkum refers to saffron, the star ingredient in the solution. Translated, the name 'kumkumadi tailam' means 'saffron and other materials, in oil.'

The traditional preparation of the kumkumadi tailam involves making a paste of saffron and rose water, adding in 26 different herbs and extracts (in specific proportions, of course), and then preserving it in a base of oil and goat milk. If that sounds like a potion straight from some mythological tale, let me tell you, the benefits it offers are no less mythical.

Saffron improves blood circulation, giving your skin that radiant glow, which is very difficult to achieve with makeup or other cosmetic cover-ups. Saffron influences your epidermal inflammatory response and breaks the chain of chemical processes that trigger the release of excess melanin—so this infusion can also be used for spot treatment of dark circles and areas that have scars, marks, or hyperpigmentation. Apart from this, saffron has antioxidant, antibacterial, antimicrobial, and anti-inflammatory properties, which prevents and treats acne, eczema, psoriasis, and so many other skin conditions for which allopathic formulations offer no cure. Saffron pollen present in kumkumadi tailam acts as a natural sunscreen, while the oil functions as a moisturizer. Maybe I should have just spoken about this in the 'all-rounder' chapter earlier! But seriously, this is as amazing an all-around performance from one single formulation as one can expect.?

While saffron oil gets absorbed into your skin pretty fast and does work as a natural illuminator, it does not promise instant results. No Ayurvedic solution does. As with all natural products, consistency is key, and it requires you to follow a regular regime before you see any results. Watch out for beauty products that claim immediate results, or even give you an exact number of days for the effects to kick in. That is usually a sign that such beauty products are chock full of harsh chemicals, even if the brand claims to be all-natural or Ayurvedic.

And here's where customization comes in. Saffron oil-based gels, serums, and creams are recommended to people of all skin types. The proportion of oil and goat milk is adjusted in a way that makes the mixture more or less oily, thereby creating a bespoke solution that caters to specific needs. And the best part? To get this kind of a customized solution elsewhere in the market, one would have to pay an eye-popping hefty price—but Ayurveda makes it more accessible to everyone.

They work by providing nourishment

One of my earliest memories is of my grandmother grabbing me by the shoulders and sitting me down on the floor in front of her chair. She would then proceed to give me a coconut oil 'champi' or head massage. I would always protest pretty loudly—the indignity of being hauled unceremoniously away from my games, only to be subjected to this vigorous action on my head! But my grandma would always patiently explain how it would enhance blood circulation in my scalp and improve the quality of my hair. (I was never too convinced back then. I would have preferred to play a little while longer before bath time.)

Of course, that wasn't my only experience with coconut oil. Coming from a pretty traditional south Indian family, I was quite familiar with it. My mother, aunts, and older cousins would all nourish their hair with it before bathing. Some of the more traditional food items in our festive thali (assorted platter) would be cooked with it. My grandfather would even apply some medicated coconut oil infused with various herbs to his joints, as it is known to ease arthritic pain. In fact, I had pretty much always taken this oil for granted.

Imagine my surprise, when a few years back, it started being hailed as the next big thing in health! Today, anybody who knows anything about health and wellness will wax lyrical about the multiple benefits of coconut oil. People across the world are now baking their cakes with it, removing their makeup with it, and even blending it into their coffee! However, the first thing I think of when someone talks about coconut oil is my grandma's soft voice assuring me that it will make my hair thick and strong.

Indeed, coconut oil has some amazingly nourishing properties that makes it a fantastic ingredient in both hair and skincare products. It contains lauric and caprylic acids, which give it antibacterial and anti-fungal properties, and its high vitamin E and healthy fat content makes it intensely nourishing. Coconut oil is invaluable for those with eczema, psoriasis, dermatitis, or other skin conditions that might result in dryness and flaking skin. It also makes for a great alternative to chemical makeup removers and forms a fabulous base for many face masks, body masks, lip scrubs, and exfoliants.

And when it comes to haircare, coconut oil has near-magical properties that put it far ahead of any other 'miracle' product you might find in the market. It deep-conditions the hair and tones the scalp. It promotes hair growth, is used in anti-dandruff treatments, and is also great for those looking to slow down premature greying. Of course, there are many oils that might prove nourishing for your hair. But the particular molecular and fatty acid structure of coconut oil allows it to penetrate the hair shaft far more easily. These benefits are not new discoveries either—just ask any Indian grandmother about haircare, and chances are, she'll recommend coconut oil just off the top of her head.

Coconut oil certainly does slow down hair fall, but it does so by nourishing your hair shaft to prevent breakage and by improving scalp health by enhancing the growth of good bacteria. However, there's one thing that even coconut oil can't defeat—and that's genetics ☺! If baldness is in your genes, then even dipping your entire head in a vat of coconut oil ain't gonna help! But for all other things associated with haircare, nothing comes close to the wonder that is coconut oil!

They work by boosting the right proteins and hormones in your body

Anti-aging products are another category of cosmetics that are in high demand today. Guess where the global market stands today, even amidst a global pandemic? The industry has a whopping $52.5 billion market in the year 2020[15]. It seems everyone and their grandmothers want a drop of the elixir of youth.

When it comes to antiaging, again, there is nothing that will stop the march of time. What cosmetic solutions can do is plump up and hydrate your skin, so that fine lines and wrinkles are not so obvious. This is how most antiaging products in the market work. The other option is to boost the right proteins in your body that help the skin repair and regenerate. Ayurveda does a bit of both—not to stop aging, but rather, to help you age gracefully.

Collagen is the one fundamental protein in our skin that enables it to maintain its shape and structural integrity. When we are young, our body naturally produces enough collagen to stay ahead of the everyday wear and tear of the skin. But as we grow older, the collagen production slows down, causing fine lines, wrinkles, and crow's feet to appear. This is when we need to boost the body to produce more collagen.

Today, collagen may be the biggest buzzword in antiaging formulas, and creams and serums containing collagen reflect this in their price tags. But the topical application of collagen is seldom very effective—the molecular structure of the protein is such that it doesn't get easily absorbed into the skin. The better alternative, then, is to stimulate and boost the production of collagen in the body. Of course, there are synthetic supplements available that can do this as well—but here again, one has to deal with side effects like heartburn, joint pain, and overproduction of calcium in the body. These supplements are also known to trigger allergies in some cases.

The Ayurvedic solutions to boost collagen in the body are generally much safer and do not have such side effects. Rather than the topical application of collagen, Ayurvedic creams and gels contain honey, coconut oil, and herbs like brahmi, horsetail, and hawthorn. These are high in antioxidants and are known to stimulate and stabilize collagen naturally.

In the chapter where we discussed nutrition, I had mentioned how important dairy products were in our day-to-day dietary requirements—

---

15 https://www.globenewswire.com/news-release/2020/07/22/2065721/0/en/Global-Anti-Aging-Products-Industry.html

and you might even remember the role they played in maternal diets. Here, dairy makes an appearance again, this time with massive benefits for the skin. Natural oils and herbs blended with milk make for great topical balms to boost collagen and hydrate and plump up the skin. Aged ghee made from cow's milk is yet another fantastic ingredient for antiaging skin balms—it nourishes, tones, and adds luster to the skin, making fine lines and wrinkles less prominent.

Let me wrap up this chapter on beauty with a nostalgic remembrance of a practice that has all but disappeared today—something that we jokingly referred to as an 'oil regime.' Basically, back in the day, if we complained to our grandparents about anything at all, they'd point us to an oil to cure it. Got dry skin? Heat a few peppercorns and fenugreek seeds in sesame oil and apply all over the body. It works as a wonderful moisturizer. Coming down with a cold or sinus? Take a few drops of mustard oil on your fingers and inhale, coating the inside of your nostrils. That cold will never come around. Feeling a tad constipated? Having a little spoonful of castor oil will do the trick. Even when the toddlers in our family would suffer from colic and griping, my grandparents would mix a bit of coconut oil with asafetida to make a paste and apply it around the navel. While we did joke and tease them about their oil regime, more often than not, these remedies worked! I guess it's true what they say—whatever your complaint, there's an oil for that! But stay away from that snake-oil salesman, though!

CHAPTER 9

International Yoga Day: Why Yoga is an Important Aspect of Ayurveda

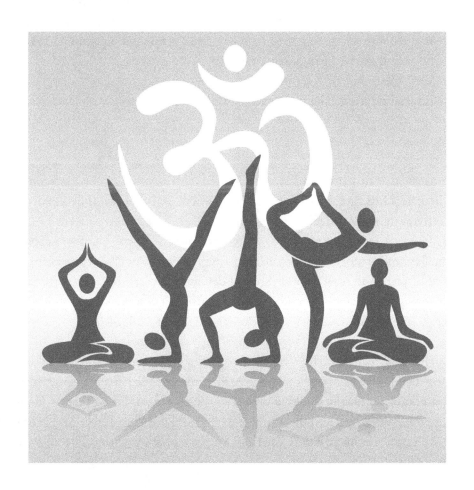

SEVERAL YEARS BACK, I was in the U.S. for a three-day conference. As it usually happens at events like these, many people who had flown in to attend the sessions were put up in the same hotel. Early on the morning of Day 2, I went downstairs to the hotel lounge to grab a quick breakfast before the sessions started. Seeing some of my fellow conference participants walk in too, I waved them over to my table.

I had met most of them the day before, so the perfunctory small talk was already out of the way. Now, in a more relaxed setting, the conversation moved on to friendlier topics, and we all started getting to know each other. One woman was quite interested to know about my work and was excited to learn more about ancient Indian health care and medicine. She had recently started getting into yoga, she informed me, and had thus developed an interest in holistic practices.

'Oh, what kind of yoga do you practice?' I asked.

'The aerial kind,' she replied.

-►◄─ ◉ ◉ ─►◄-

To those as uninitiated as I was back then, this is not a cliched reference to levitation! Rather, it is a form of yoga where you practice the asanas on hammocks suspended from the ceiling.

This is just one of the many different kinds of 'yoga' out there today. Don't get me wrong—I'm not about to get into a debate about the authenticity of yoga and how nobody should deviate from the one true practice. In fact, given that so many sages and gurus have practiced and taught yoga for centuries, there isn't just one 'right' path to follow. As long as the essence of the practice is maintained, some variations are inevitable.

However, some of the strains of yoga that exist today are really taking it too far. Did you know that there's something called Beer Yoga, which apparently merges asanas with a brewery experience? And then there is Goat Yoga, Tantrum Yoga, and the ultimate oxymoron, the Yoga Rave. And here I thought practices like Bikram Yoga and Yogalate (that's yoga and Pilates) were pretty far out!

Now, of course, each of these practices has vehement defenders who'll argue that these forms make yoga more fun and accessible to the general public. And that's where I make the first interjection—I think the traditional kinds of yoga are pretty accessible, to begin with. In fact, they may even be more accessible and doable than these new-fangled varieties.

So, what is yoga, really?

Traditional yoga doesn't require any fancy equipment, expensive outfits, or even an extravagant membership to an eye-wateringly chic yoga studio. It doesn't ask you to hang from the ceiling or sweat it out in an uncomfortably hot room while you struggle to keep up with the rest of the class. In fact, it tells you to do just the opposite—sit in a clean, quiet place, be as comfortable as possible, and go at a pace that works for you.

For although most people today know yoga by its physical forms of exercise, it is actually a system that is extremely holistic. Although these days it is seen to be separate from Ayurveda, the two systems are intrinsically linked with strong roots in the Vedas. In Sanskrit, the word 'yoga' has several meanings. Let me give you a similar example in the English language. Take the word 'fair' for example. The word 'fair' has a few meanings when used as different parts of speech. When used as an adjective, it can describe someone as agreeable, but it can also describe someone who has light skin or hair. As a noun, a 'fair' is typically a local event that celebrates a certain person, place, or historical moment. The meaning one would ascribe to the word is entirely context dependent. English has quite a few such homonyms. In fact, one of the fascinating aspects of the Sanskrit language is that each word has three meanings—guhya (the hidden meaning), samadhi (that which is buried under the surface), and drishya (the obvious or the apparent one). Sometimes more than three meanings. Perhaps the most relevant meaning we could apply for the word yoga in this context would be 'to unite.' It helps unite one's mind, body, and spirit in perfect harmony. And in doing so, it also helps unite one's individual consciousness to the cosmic universe as a whole. Needless to say, that cannot happen in conjunction with loud music or distracting gimmicks.

But that is not to say that you cannot do yoga unless you are in some silent ashram and have several hours to devote to the practice every day. You can absolutely try practicing yoga in your own home, a park, or a garden. You just need to make sure that the environment is peaceful and comfortable rather than loud and hot. The early morning hours or the time around dusk are preferable, but there is no hard and fast rule about the timings. However, you do need to ensure that you do it on an empty stomach, so wait at least three–four hours after eating. The movements should be gentle and fluid rather than fast and vigorous. The ultimate goal, after all, is to achieve peace and oneness, and not to work off carbs.

In fact, in many cases, the different asanas of yoga are even interwoven into our day-to-day lives. For instance, if you attend any puja or a traditional festival in India, you might partake of the prasadam (religious offerings of food) afterward. You will notice that the worshippers and other attendees do not eat at a table—rather, they sit down cross-legged on the floor. This pose is called the sukhasana, and sitting this way during meals is extremely beneficial for health. With the plate kept on the floor in front of you, this pose automatically makes you lean forward to take every mouthful of food, and then swing back again as you chew. This back-and-forth movement aids digestion, as it promotes the secretion of your stomach enzymes. This pose also helps you realize when you are full faster, which means you can avoid overeating. Moreover, it stretches and strengthens your back, hips, and knees. Eating this way was the traditional practice in India for centuries. Today, the practice is all but lost, and only a few households still follow it, including mine.

The Four Paths of Yoga

Wondering how varied yoga really is? Let me explain. Given that people have different tastes, preferences, natures, and predispositions, it is unreasonable to expect that everyone's journey to unity and self-awareness will look the same. The practice of yoga does take that into account, and according to traditional yogic philosophy, there are four major paths that can help you achieve the same goal.

1. **Raja yoga:** This is the path that most of us are familiar with. It involves the physical poses and asanas, the pranayama breathing techniques, and the various kinds of meditation that you might be recommended.
2. **Karma yoga:** This is the path where work and selfless service to others is considered to be the journey to achieving enlightenment. Specifically, this refers to the kind of work one does for the good of others, without any expectations of payment, praise, or returns.
3. **Bhakti yoga:** This is the more devotional path that focuses on worship, faith, rituals, and service to divinity. This path, thus, tends to be more spiritual and has strong connections to religion.
4. **Jnana yoga:** This is a more philosophical path that embraces will, learning, and intellect to move away from ignorance and strive for knowledge. Those with a logical bent of mind find an affinity to this path.

Even when it comes to the path of raja yoga, which most of us are familiar with, there is no one right way to practice asanas and meditation. Different sages and rishis prescribed different ways to embrace the system.

For instance, there is Ashtanga yoga, which is an ancient eight-fold approach from the *Yoga Sutras*. The *Yoga Sutras* is a comprehensive handbook of guidelines written close to 2,000 years ago. It is usually attributed to Sage Patanjali—however, not much is known about the sage, and it is believed that this may have been the contributed work of several rishis (sages) together. The eight limbs of Ashtanga yoga encompass one's moral code, personal hygiene, asanas or postures, breathing techniques, meditation, and so on until one has managed to achieve the state of ultimate bliss.

Hatha yoga is another ancient approach that sets out guidelines for mastering and purifying one's physical and mental energies. It includes physical asanas, breathing techniques, mental and physical detoxification tactics, as well as methods to control one's thoughts and energies.

Irrespective of which path one follows or which exact approach one chooses, the ultimate goal is the same—that of achieving individual harmony and unity with the universe. Although these paths and approaches may all seem quite distinctive, regular followers know that there is a lot of overlap in the thoughts and philosophies of each system.

And likewise, there are a lot of common hindrances and disruptions that can interrupt or deviate one from the path of unity and bliss. In Ashtanga yoga, for instance, nine such disturbances are listed out:

Disease
This, of course, is the most obvious disturbance that stands in the way of us achieving our ultimate potential. Diseases of the body and the mind seep us of our strength and make us weak and uncomfortable. This prevents us from being able to focus our attention on even the simplest task at hand, let alone the lofty goal of attaining spirituality and oneness. Consistent practice of yoga is known to be a great way to stay fit and healthy, and this is the most common reason why most people embrace it today.

Laziness
All of us face this obstacle at some point or the other in our day-to-day life. Think of hitting the snooze button, sleeping in for an extra hour even when you're well-rested, or putting off a task for later. And the consequences for these are pretty immediate—giving in to laziness often means that we are rushed off our feet later, trying to juggle multiple tasks and unable to do anything well. This is yet another obstacle that yoga aims to help us overcome.

Languor
This may be closely related to laziness, but it refers to the mental aspect of our inaction. Ever had a long list of chores to do, but found yourself feeling lethargic and quite unable to get up and tackle those tasks? Then you'll know exactly what languor is. Mental inertia and languor are other obstacles that we need to overcome in order to enjoy the true potential that yoga unlocks.

Worldliness

When we get caught up in the little things, we tend to focus too much on external factors, without devoting enough time or attention to looking inwards. Self-reflection and self-awareness are important aspects of yoga, and worldliness can be a major obstacle to that.

Carelessness

This refers to those times when one has the knowledge of the correct strategies and processes—but does not pay enough attention to actually follow them. Yoga is a practice that requires precision and concentration, so carelessness can prove to be a significant obstacle.

Doubt

Doubt holds us back from achieving our full potential more than inability ever will. Have you noticed how people with mediocre skills go so far ahead by sheer force of determination, while talented people get left behind? This is true in our everyday life, and it becomes even more relevant when we're talking about loftier goals like self-actualization and inner peace.

Discouragement

The practice of yoga and the journey to achieving one's potential are experienced differently by different people. While some may see immediate results, others may need to embrace the philosophy for a lot longer before noticing any differences. Comparing your journey to someone else's is the easiest way to get discouraged.

Hallucination

This refers to the way one interprets one's experiences while practicing a spiritual system like yoga. Misinterpretation and misunderstanding of one's experiences can hamper one's progress and hinder one's journey to reaching one's potential.

Instability

This basically refers to inconsistency. Whether we're talking about the physical challenges of practicing yoga or the mental strength needed to control one's thoughts and emotions, stability is key to moving on to one's higher self. Being inconsistent and irregular gets in the way of that, and proves to be a major obstacle.

Yoga and its Therapeutic Properties

Now let's come to the role of yoga in healing and health care. As we have seen in the previous chapters, Ayurveda aims for holistic well-being, and exercise and fitness are very important aspects of that. This is where yoga's link to Ayurveda becomes more apparent.

Yoga has been used for centuries to balance one's doshas and keep the body healthy, flexible, and free of diseases. In recent years, the healing properties of yoga have become more well-known too. And just like you can choose your yogic approach based on your predispositions and nature, it is also possible to choose the right kind of yoga as per your physical and medical needs.

Yoga based on doshas

Here's yet another reason to choose traditional yoga practices over the more trendy and gimmicky versions. In modern yoga classes or group sessions, the trainers take you through a set sequence, and you're expected to keep up. In traditional methods, however, you might be prescribed a more personalized sequence based on your dosha or physical constitution. Certain asanas may work better for you as they balance your dosha rather than aggravating it.

- **Vata dosha:** If you have a vata dominant body type, you might need exercises that are more grounding and fluid. The yoga poses that will be prescribed to you, thus, would focus on the lower half of your body and put pressure on your hips and pelvis—maybe something like the balasana (child's pose) or dhanurasana (bow pose). You might also find it more calming to take on more meditative asanas like padmasana (lotus pose), virasana (hero pose), or even the savasana (corpse pose). When it comes to pranayama, those with vata body types are generally asked to avoid the more cooling or overly stimulating breathing techniques like sitali or kapalabhati.

- **Pitta dosha:** Intensity and fiery spirits mark out those with pitta dominant body types. Calming and soothing yoga poses that focus on one's chest and abdomen are considered to be ideal for those with a pitta metabolism. Think of the ustrasana (camel pose) that stretches your chest, back, and solar plexus, bhujangasana (cobra pose) that dissipates aggression and energy or ardha matsyendrasana (half lord-of-fishes pose) that twists the abdomen. Cooling pranayamas like sitali are perfect for those with this body type.
- **Kapha dosha:** Characteristics like heaviness, sluggishness, and compact density define those of the kapha metabolic category. Warming and stimulating yoga poses will most likely be recommended to those of kapha constitution, and the main focus will be on the chest and upper abdomen. Asanas that bend the back, like salabhasana (locust pose), setu bandhasana (bridge pose), and ustrasana (camel pose) would be ideal. As for pranayama, stimulating and warming breathing techniques like kapalbhati or ujjayi are recommended.

Of course, these are just the basic principles of practicing yoga based on one's dosha. A licensed practitioner will take several other factors into account, like your age, environment, season, medical restrictions, and so on. But the key, ultimately, is to find a sequence that works for you, rather than opting for more generic sessions.

Yoga as a healing practice
Apart from helping you keep your mind and body healthy and preventing various illnesses and ailments, yoga holds a significant position in treatment

and medical care too. Ayurvedic practitioners are likely to suggest certain yoga therapies to work alongside the medicines they prescribe. So, what kind of diseases and ailments can yoga help cure? Let's take a look.

1. **Cardiovascular conditions**

   We already know that those suffering from heart conditions and cardiovascular diseases often have various lifestyle-driven factors like stress, hypertension, high cholesterol, and obesity playing into them. Any Ayurvedic practitioner will look at tackling these issues urgently, rather than just prescribing medication. We have already seen how these issues are managed through good dietary habits. When it comes to exercise, yoga can be a great option in helping the patient move to a healthier, more sustainable lifestyle. It helps strengthen the muscles, brings down one's BMI, and decreases the markers of inflammation, all of which are instrumental in keeping your heart healthy.

   Of course, any form of exercise is beneficial, but yoga has some extra benefits that you don't get by just going for a run. Yoga's grounding techniques and mindful breathing practices have a perceptible impact in lowering stress and managing anxiety. This, in turn, brings down your blood pressure. What's more, stress also has an indirect link to cholesterol. Those suffering from chronic stress and anxiety tend to generate high levels of cortisol and adrenaline, which basically means that your body is constantly in fight-or-flight mode. This prompts your body to store triglycerides in your fat cells— which may result in increased levels of bad cholesterol and eventual hardening of the arteries. Managing stress through yoga thus can help reverse these conditions—and if you practice it already, it may prevent these eventualities from arising in the first place.

   In addition to these, yoga has also been found to have a positive impact on those suffering from atrial fibrillation. This is a condition that is marked by irregular and abnormally fast heartbeats. Though it is quite common, this is a serious ailment. Left unchecked, atrial fibrillation (or AFib) episodes can worsen and can even lead to strokes or heart failure. Yoga is often recommended to AFib patients as it is gentle enough to be practiced without putting any additional strain on the heart. In fact, one study recently found that simply going through the standard treatment for AFib was not nearly as effective as taking medication while also practicing yoga. Yoga was seen to bring down the frequency of AFib episodes and stabilize the heartbeat.

2. **Musculoskeletal disorders**

If your job requires you to sit in front of a computer all day, chances are, you lead a sedentary lifestyle. Sitting for long hours (especially if your posture happens to be poor) affects your musculoskeletal structure in a variety of ways—it causes the pelvis to tilt forward, puts pressure on your spine, and shortens the hip flexors, to name a few issues. If you experience joint pain and chronic ache in your lower back, shoulders, and neck, you are already noticing the fallouts.

Yoga has been known to undo a lot of these issues. It offers a safe way to work out your muscles with minimal risk of injuries. It helps strengthen your muscles, stretches out the ones that have become shortened or tightened over time, and releases tension. These, in turn, reduce stress on your joints, bones, and ligaments. Moreover, yoga also helps regulate your synovial fluid, which keeps your joints well lubricated. Studies have noted that those suffering from lower back pain report reduced pain intensity and regained mobility faster once they start doing yoga.

Yoga also has significant benefits when it comes to graver musculoskeletal concerns. Take osteoarthritis, for instance. This is a common joint condition that comes from the wear and tear of the cartilage. Regular exercise and movement of the joints are mandatory in managing and treating the condition. In a cruel twist of fate, the slightest movement can cause pain to those suffering from osteoarthritis—leaving them fairly disinclined to exercise. The gentler forms of yoga are the ideal solution here and poses like tadagasana (pond pose), vajrasana (thunderbolt pose), and vrikshasana (tree pose) can easily be adopted even by beginners. Regular yoga has been shown to reduce pain intensity and improve mobility and range.

Likewise, yoga has also been widely used to enhance bone mass and relieve symptoms of disorders like osteoporosis, multiple sclerosis, and carpal tunnel syndrome. Apart from the purely physical benefits, yogic breathing and relaxation techniques can help manage pain and anxiety where even medication fails.

3. **Endocrine disorders**

Quick question: How often have you experienced fatigue, random mood swings, sudden weight gain, general sluggishness, irregular menstrual cycles, headaches, body cramps, and a high frequency of colds and flus?

Next question: When was the last time you actually went to a doctor for any of these issues?

Unfortunately, most of us face at least some of these issues regularly, but we consider them as nothing out of the ordinary. After all, we already know that these are results of a poor lifestyle. You may realize that your cramps, headaches, and insomnia are results of all that extra stress from that new project at work. Or that your sedentary lifestyle has caused your metabolism to slow down and your periods to go haywire. But given that the triggers (stress, a desk job, poor diet) are not going anywhere, we often dismiss the results as 'normal.' However, these are some of the most common signs of your hormones being in disarray.

The endocrine system is made up of all the glands that produce and regulate hormones in our body. Environmental and lifestyle-led factors can impact these glands, leading to the production of too much or too little of these hormones. This disbalance is what causes all these constant niggling issues. Now, most of us fully intend to fix our lifestyle—eat healthy, exercise, get enough sleep. But these are massive lifestyle changes, so we keep putting them off. That's again where yoga can come in and save the day.

Certain asanas stimulate or relax particular glands, which can be instrumental in balancing out the hormones produced by that gland.

For example, the dhanurasana (bow pose) stimulates the adrenal gland, the halasana (plow pose) works the thyroid gland, and the sirsasana (headstand) stimulates the pineal and pituitary glands. In this way, a yoga routine that targets specific glands can be the most effective way to bring your endocrine system back in sync and improve your general health.

Those suffering from serious endocrine disorders like PCOS have reported massive benefits from yoga practices. Not only does yoga help them lose weight, but it also helps reduce testosterone, anti-Müllerian hormone, and luteinizing hormone levels in the body. This helps tackle many of the fallouts of PCOS. Likewise, yoga has also been successfully used to control insulin production in the body, thereby helping manage type-2 diabetes. These are just some of the more common endocrine disorders that yoga can help you with. With the right kinds of asanas, combined with the right medication and dietary changes, the possibilities are endless.

4. **Respiratory health**

Asthma, allergies, and shortness of breath are daily complaints for a lot of people—especially if they reside in the more polluted cities. Pollen, dust, smoke, and fibers can trigger severe allergies and breathing disorders in those who suffer from these conditions. But here again, these patients don't think these are anything out of the ordinary—they have long since resigned themselves to the fact that these disorders are 'incurable.' However, just controlling the symptoms is not the ideal solution. Now, especially in light of the Covid-19 pandemic, we are fast waking up to the true importance of proper lung functioning.

A few chapters back, we discussed how Ayurveda can (and does) offer permanent cures for allergies and breathing disorders. But aside from medicines, your Ayurvedic practitioner may suggest some regular yoga exercises and practices to supplement the treatment.

Yoga, after all, has a profound effect on respiratory health. When done right, even the most basic asanas help you alter your breathing patterns—they stretch out your lungs, forcing you to take deeper breaths, and then compress them, thereby making you exhale fully. Many asanas also help strengthen the diaphragm and thoracic muscles, which further help in improving respiratory health. Then there are certain yogic practices or kriyas like nasal irrigation and oil pulling, which may help expel mucus, phlegm, and other secretions. This keeps the respiratory passages clean. And of course, the special pranayama breathing techniques also go a long way in regulating and controlling your lung function.

Studies have shown that a combination of these techniques, together with the right medicines, do actually work wonders. Asthma patients, for instance, exhibit improved pulmonary parameters when they regularly practice yoga. They are not as easily triggered by common irritants; their asthmatic episodes are often less severe, and they need to resort to rescue medication much less frequently than before. Those with permanent lung damage from conditions like chronic bronchitis, emphysema, and other chronic obstructive pulmonary diseases (COPD), have been found to be able to manage their symptoms better with regular yoga.

Moreover, these disorders often have a mental component to them too, which aggravates the breathing difficulties. This sparks off a vicious cycle—the stress exacerbates bronchial constriction, which in turn causes more stress and panic. Yoga helps manage the stress symptoms that are associated with breathing difficulties too.

5. Pregnancy

Strong muscles, a healthy heart, and great mental health are always important—but especially so during pregnancy. Ironically, this is the one time when a woman might be most hesitant to maintain a regular workout routine. At a stage when you'd like to keep the strenuous physical activity to a minimum, yoga offers a calming and safe alternative to take care of your health without putting your baby at risk. Do run it by your doctor first, of course—and it's also best to seek guidance from a licensed yoga practitioner who specializes in prenatal training. They will be able to craft a personalized yoga routine that guides you through every trimester.

Women who do yoga regularly before and during pregnancy, experience fewer aches and pains. This is because the right asanas help tone and develop the right set of muscles at a time when their bodies are changing almost on a weekly basis. Yoga improves blood circulation, enhances digestion, and stretches out your muscles, thereby allaying other pregnancy-related physical discomforts like nausea, breathlessness, swollen ankles, and headaches.

The mental and emotional benefits of yoga during pregnancy cannot be ignored either. Yoga has been shown to lower the levels of perceived stress in an expecting mother—which is extremely important, given that hypertension and stress can have negative effects on the baby. Sukha pranayama, a special yogic breathing technique, has actually been found to have positive impacts on heart rate and blood pressure with near immediate effect (we're talking within five minutes!). These benefits extend from the mother to the baby if practiced during pregnancy.

Another great reason to make yoga a regular part of your pregnancy wellness routine? It strengthens your hip muscles, core, and pelvic floor—all of which are going to result in an easier delivery. Women who practiced yoga during their pregnancy were noted to have shorter labor, especially during the first stage. When asked to evaluate their labor pain during and after delivery, they reported higher levels of maternal comfort. Plus, those who are familiar with the practice of pranayama are already trained to breathe deeply and more mindfully. This obviously proves indispensable during those crucial hours when your breathing technique is your most important tool to relax and loosen your muscles.

6. **Mental health**

So far, we have only discussed mental health in relation to other diseases and disorders. Sure, yoga can reduce stress, panic, and anxiety, which automatically leads to a whole host of benefits for the different systems in your body. But what if you are looking for a therapeutic tool to manage certain mental health symptoms on your own? Can yoga help with that?

The answer is a resounding yes. The therapeutic benefits of yoga have been well documented when it comes to various mental health issues—from the more common anxiety and depressive disorders, going right up to more severe forms of autism, and even schizophrenia.

Yoga can guide you to a deep state of neurobiological relaxation. This is a state of calmness and rest that cannot be achieved by any other relaxing activities like, say, watching a movie or talking to a friend. These activities still require some level of mental and social engagement that keeps your brain quite pumped up. After all, you do need to pay enough attention to follow the plot of that movie or respond to whatever your friend just said. But yoga doesn't require any responses to external stimuli—instead, it helps power down the adrenaline and the other chemical reactions. In essence, yoga's deep breathing patterns enable you to move from your sympathetic nervous system (the fight-or-flight state) to your parasympathetic nervous system (the rest-and-digest state).

Those suffering from anxiety and depressive disorders typically record low levels of a particular brain chemical called gamma-amino-butyric acid or GABA. This is the chemical that inhibits neural activity. Low levels of this chemical imply that your neurotransmitters do not slow down, resulting in jitteriness, restlessness, and anxious thought loops. Yoga has been shown to increase GABA levels way more than other physical and mental activities like walking or reading. Needless to say, this has immense benefits for those looking to manage anxiety, depression, or panic disorders.

Yoga therapies have been successful in treating specific mental disorders and learning disabilities too. Such therapies have been shown to have positive effects on attention deficit disorder (ADD)/ ADHD—one study actually showed a 91 percent reduction in symptoms. They have also been found to ease the symptoms of autism in kids, resulting in improved coordination, flexibility, social responses, and communication skills. These kinds of functional yoga therapies have proven to be a boon for parents of kids with special needs everywhere.

What's more, the benefits of yoga therapy even extend to those suffering from eating disorders and addictions. Used in conjunction with drug intervention, it has shown positive results for treating psychotic disorders too.

-»≡◉ ◉≡«-

This brings me to the end of this book. Of course, a compendium, it is not! These nine chapters have merely scratched the surface of the wealth of information that Ayurveda provides. But I do hope that I have been able to dispel some myths and misconceptions and clear up some misunderstandings about Ayurveda that are widespread today.

I hope:

- You now have a better idea of what Ayurveda is—as well as what it's not!
- You are able to understand that there are solutions in Ayurveda for many diseases and conditions that allopathy is not able to fix or if it does, it leads to several nasty side effects.
- When it comes to immunity, you are able to appreciate that Ayurveda is a time-tested methodology and system that can promote wellness. Ironically enough, while immunity is a concept popularized by allopathy, Western science has already started looking towards India and Ayurveda to build a strong immune system.
- You are able to appreciate that COVID-19 has been successfully treated with Ayurveda. Thousands of patients have been cured and have made strong recoveries by adopting the Ayurvedic treatment regimen. This is both inexpensive as well as safe.

- That the next time someone panics about the 'hard metals' in Ayurvedic preparations, or talks about all the restrictions that an Ayurvedic lifestyle involves—you are able to tell them otherwise.
- That the next time you come across an influencer talking about another life-changing diet or a brand-new superfood, you are able to weigh its legitimacy in a more logical, rational way.
- That when yet another magazine markets yet another cosmetic product as an expensive 'must-have,' you are inspired to find a cheaper, better, and more effective natural alternative.
- That when you come across a one-size-fits-all solution, you are able to look at it with some suspicion and probe deeper into those claims.

Above all, I hope that some of the information in this book helps you lead a more balanced, happier, healthier life.

CPSIA information can be obtained
at www.ICGtesting.com
Printed in the USA
BVHW041333230721
612717BV00012B/461

9 789390 976782